return or
t at
our free

the new
eat for life

By the same author:

Eat for Life Diet
Ultimate Ace Diet
Healthy Eating on a Plate
The Really Useful Teenage Food Diet

the new
eat
for
life

A revolutionary new eating and exercise plan
based on the ground-breaking findings of the
World Health Organisation

Janette Marshall

Vermilion
LONDON

1 3 5 7 9 10 8 6 4 2

First published in 2003 by Vermilion,
an imprint of Ebury Press, Random House,
20 Vauxhall Bridge Road, London SW1V 2SA
www.randomhouse.co.uk

Random House Australia (Pty) Limited
20 Alfred Street, Milsons Point, Sydney,
New South Wales 2061, Australia

Random House New Zealand Limited
18 Poland Road, Glenfield,
Auckland 10, New Zealand

Random House South Africa (Pty) Limited
Endulini, 5A Jubilee Road,
Parktown 2193, South Africa

The Random House Group Limited Reg. No. 954009

A CIP catalogue record for this book
is available from the British Library

ISBN 0-09-189458-1

Penguin Random House is committed to a sustainable future for
our business, our readers and our planet. This book is made from
Forest Stewardship Council® certified paper.

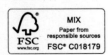

Printed and bound in Great Britain by Clays Ltd, Elcograf S.p.A.

WARNING

If you have a medical condition, or are
pregnant, the diet or exercises
described in this book should not be
followed without first consulting your
doctor. All guidelines and warnings
should be read carefully, and the
author and publisher cannot accept
responsibility for injuries or damage
arising out of a failure to comply with
the same.

CONTENTS

Chapter 1
One diet fits all

The biggest epidemic of disease in the world today is largely preventable. It affects both developed and developing countries. You can't catch it as you might a cold, measles or smallpox, but it is catching in the sense that as the developing world adopts a Western diet and lifestyle, the global epidemic increases.

PROTECT YOURSELF FROM THE GLOBAL EPIDEMIC

The epidemic that is sweeping the world is not just one disease – it's a whole host of chronic (long-term) diseases that are disabling and miserable to the individuals they affect, and disastrous to society because they cost so much to treat. It is estimated that 46 per cent of the burden of disease in the world today is due to these non-communicable diseases.

Scientists have known for a long time that diseases such as cancer and heart disease are largely preventable, and now they have proof that the causes are:
• the wrong diet
• too little physical activity
• smoking
• over-consumption of alcohol

For the first time in human history the world's total of overweight people equals the total of those who are underfed. More than 1 billion eat more than they need, and as many go hungry each day.

This book is concerned with the health problems created by excess. All over the world, including some developing countries, people are eating more calories than they need, particularly in the form of saturated fats. They are also not getting enough vitamins, minerals and other protective substances in food.

Eating too much, combined with a sedentary lifestyle, is causing more and more people to die prematurely or be disabled by obesity and other health problems, such as type 2 diabetes, cancer, heart disease, high blood pressure, stroke and osteoporosis. All these

ONE SMALL STEP...

The worldwide problem of obesity appears daunting, but even small changes can help over time. For example, cutting out one biscuit a day (or buying a smaller burger than usual) and walking 1.6 km (1 mile) a day could 'save' you 100 calories. That's enough to prevent the annual 1 kg/2 lb weight gain that happens to most adults and that can eventually lead to obesity.

conditions cause individual misery and a huge burden on health and social budgets.

WHAT CAN YOU DO?

Choosing the right balance of food, being more active and giving up smoking are the most significant things you can do to help prevent or reduce the number of unhealthy years you live with long-term disabling health problems. More importantly, altering diet and increasing physical activity can improve your quality of life so that you feel healthier, happier and more positive about your future and that of your children.

Diet and lifestyle changes should be priorities for every individual not only because heart disease, obesity and type 2 diabetes are growing at an alarming rate, but because they are now appearing earlier in life and threatening to affect children. At the other end of the life span they cause costly disabilities in the elderly, which take a heavy toll on their families and the State.

It is estimated that by the year 2020 almost three-quarters of deaths in the world will be due to these largely preventable diseases. Around 70 per cent of the deaths will be from heart disease, stroke and type 2 diabetes in both the developed and developing worlds. But in the developing world, the diseases of 'over-nutrition' will be overtaking the diseases of under-nutrition within 20 years. Already lifestyle-related heart disease is spreading through India and China, and obesity is a serious problem in Latin America and parts of Africa, where it co-exists with hunger and malnutrition.

We might not understand all the scientific minutiae of how diet relates to health, but there is a mountain of plausible science in place to show what we can do to reduce the risks to our health. This book will set you in the right direction.

BREAKING FREE OF THE STATISTICS

Making healthier choices is not always easy. A culture dominated by ready-made and fast food, lack of time and sedentary occupations means you must make an effort to reject unhealthy norms, including smoking, overeating and more than moderate alcohol intake.

With more than 1 billion smokers in the world, 1 billion people who are overweight and countless millions of people with often undiag-nosed high blood pressure, high cholesterol levels and type 2 diabetes, it might seem too late to change, but it's not. By making healthier choices you can prevent yourself from becoming one of these statistics, and in many instances reverse these health problems if you already have them.

MAKE CHANGE WORK FOR YOU

It is remarkable what can be achieved by changing bad habits: 90 per cent of all type 2 diabetes, 80 per cent of all coronary heart disease, and 30 per cent of all cancers can be avoided by making some straightforward changes to your life.

You can change: what you eat, how much physical activity you take, how much alcohol you drink, and whether you smoke. You might also be able to influence your family and friends for the better, or ask them to support you. Perhaps you could alter your home or environment to make them healthier.

You can't change: your age, gender and genetic make-up, but you can alter your diet and lifestyle to reduce your risk of diseases to which you are genetically susceptible.

If you think this doesn't apply to you because your current weight or activity level has not yet resulted in any symptoms of disease, think again. Market research shows that most people think 'It will never happen to me', that it is going to be someone else's problem – a neighbour, a colleague or another person in the family. The reality is that we are talking about *you*. Many chronic diseases have no visible signs until you suffer your first heart attack or the side-effects of high blood pressure. All the more reason to adopt a healthy, preventive diet and lifestyle.

Being overweight can shorten your life

At 20 an obese man can expect his life to be 13 years shorter than that of a normal-weight contemporary, and an obese woman of the same age may have her life expectancy cut by eight years.

At 40 an obese man loses six years of life, and an obese woman seven years. Being overweight rather than obese at 40 shortens life expectancy by around three years.

Overweight smokers are likely to die around 13 years before their non-smoking counterparts.

OUTWITTING YOUR GENES

A sense of fatalism and powerlessness in the face of your genetic inheritance might make change seem pointless or futile; in most cases it's not. Your genes might mean that you are more susceptible to diabetes than your best friend, but if your friend opts for an unhealthy, sedentary lifestyle and you take the healthier option, he or she might end up with type 2 diabetes, and you might never have it, or have it for fewer years.

Similarly, if you have a genetic predisposition to osteoarthritis or another auto-immune disease, a healthy diet rich in omega-3 fats (from oily fish, for example) might lower high levels of body chemicals associated with the condition.

A tendency to high cholesterol levels can often be helped with diet and exercise. (However, a family predisposition towards very high cholesterol levels requires drugs and diet to control it.)

In the majority of cases, therefore, your genes do not mean that a heart attack or stroke are inevitable, or that your health is definitely going to suffer. Neither (except in a few rare cases) can genetic make-up be used as a reason for being overweight or obese. The epidemic of weight problems and obesity spans just the last few decades, and genes have not changed that quickly. Yes, there are genes that switch fat cell formation on and off, that influence appetite and that make it harder or easier to lose weight, but they cannot cancel out the benefits of a healthy diet and active lifestyle.

Some people blame their weight problems on other causes outside their control, such as:

Thyroid problems – but an underactive thyroid gland accounts for a maximum of only around 5 kg/11 lb of extra weight.

Polycystic ovarian syndrome – a hormone imbalance, usually resulting in multiple cysts on the ovaries, but again weight problems associated with it can be improved by diet and exercise.

Prescription drugs – while medication for mental health problems or epilepsy, oral contraceptives and corticosteroids can all cause weight gain, it can be managed to a certain extent by diet and exercise.

Even if your genetic inheritance means it is virtually inevitable that you will suffer a particular chronic disease, you can delay it through diet and lifestyle. As we face longer lives, it becomes more important to put off (or, ideally, avoid completely) disabling health conditions. After all, a longer life is not desirable if it involves years of disability and dependence on others.

NEVER TOO OLD

Don't think you can get away with saying you are too old to benefit from change. It's never too late to adopt healthy habits. Older people with high blood pressure, for example, can change their diet and (under supervision in some cases) become more active to reduce their blood pressure and reliance on medications.

Even if you have already suffered some damage, such as developing type 2 diabetes, changing your diet and increasing your level of activity may be all it takes to put the condition into reverse. Similarly, higher than desirable levels of blood cholesterol can usually be lowered by changes to diet and becoming more active.

TOBACCO IS BAD NEWS

Smoking has a huge impact on increasing the risk of chronic disease. For example, it quadruples the risk of stroke, and, when combined with high blood pressure, the risk increases eightfold. Smoking is also the most common cause of cancer.

Unfortunately, smoking is mistakenly used as a way of controlling appetite and therefore weight gain. While weight control is important in preventing chronic disease, it cannot justify smoking as a slimming aid because it has far too many other health risks.

It is a fallacy that smoking helps weight loss. While it might suppress appetite and increase

ARE YOU AT RISK?

HEALTH FACTOR	WARNING SIGNS	INCREASED RISKS
High blood pressure	Systolic pressure (the top number in a blood pressure reading) higher than 140 mm Hg (see pages 24–25).	Heart disease, stroke and other cardio-vascular problems. *Probably also contributes to renal (kidney) failure.*
High cholesterol	Total blood cholesterol higher than 5.0 mmol/l (see page 27).	Heart disease and stroke. *Probably also contributes to other cardiovascular problems.*
Excess weight	Body mass index (BMI) greater than 25 in adults. Obesity is a BMI of 30. *See page 18 to calculate your own BMI.*	Heart disease, stroke, diabetes, osteo-arthritis, cancer of the colon and endometrium, post-menopausal breast cancer. *Probably also contributes to gall bladder cancer, kidney cancer, breathlessness, back pain, dermatitis, menstrual disorders, infertility, gallstones.*

Source: Adapted from 'Selected Major Risk Factors and Global and Regional Burdens of Disease', *The Lancet*, Vol. 360, pages 1347–60 (2002). Reprinted with permission from Elsevier.

the metabolic rate (the speed at which calories are used), the effect is short-lived.

Having started to smoke, some people are reluctant to give up because they fear getting fat. Weight gain, however, is not inevitable. Initially the metabolic rate shows down, but increasing physical activity and making the right food choices soon sees any small weight gain disappear.

There are many health and social benefits to giving up smoking:
- After 20 minutes your blood pressure and pulse rate begin to return to normal, and the circulation in your hands and feet improves.
- After 24 hours the nicotine has left your body, and your lungs begin to clear out mucus and debris.
- After 72 hours your breathing becomes easier and energy levels increase.
- After one week you will notice that there is more money in your pocket and that your hair and clothes don't smell of smoke.
- After three to nine months coughing and shortness of breath subside, and overall lung function will have improved by 5–10 per cent.
- After one year the risk of heart disease is halved, and a 20-a-day quitter will have saved more than £1500.
- After five years the risk of having a heart attack falls to about half that of a smoker.
- After 10 years the risk of lung cancer falls to around half that of a smoker. The risk of a heart attack falls to about the same as someone who has never smoked. The risk of fracture from osteoporosis becomes similar to that of lifelong non-smokers.

If you would like help to stop smoking, contact one of the following helplines:
Quitline 0800 00 22 00
NHS Smoking Helpline 0800 169 0 169
NHS Pregnancy Smoking Helpline
0800 169 9 169

WHAT'S THE POINT OF CHANGING YOUR WAYS?

The pay-off for leading a healthier life is a longer life, but – more importantly – one that has less chance of being dogged by chronic illness, notably during the last years. The table (right) shows that we in the UK have some way to go to meet the average healthy life expectancy of Japan, which tops the table with an average of 74.5 years. This figure is based on the number of years that both men and women might expect to live in full health, not the number of years they might live in total. In Japan the healthy life expectancy is 77.2 years for women and 71.9 for men, which gives an average of 74.5.

In most countries women live about four years longer than men. The widest discrepancy between the sexes is in Russia, where healthy life expectancy is 66.4 years for women but just 56.1 for men. Similar rates exist in other countries of the former Soviet Union, such as Latvia, Estonia, Belarus and Kazakhstan. In the Middle East and North Africa, on the other hand, there is less discrepancy between the sexes. Saudi Arabia, for example, has a healthy life expectancy of 65.1 for men compared with 64.0 for women. (In sub-Saharan Africa, where HIV-AIDS is prevalent, the population has a tragically low life expectancy of less than 35 years.)

HEALTHY LIFE EXPECTANCY

World Ranking	Country	Years
1	Japan	74.5
2	Australia	73.2
3	France	73.1
4	Sweden	73.0
5	Spain	72.8
6	Italy	72.7
7	Greece	72.5
8	Switzerland	72.5
9	Monaco	72.4
10	Andorra	72.3
11	San Marino	72.3
12	Canada	72.0
13	Netherlands	72.0
14	**United Kingdom**	**71.7**
15	Norway	71.7
16	Belgium	71.6
17	Austria	71.6
18	Luxembourg	71.1
19	Iceland	70.8
20	Finland	70.5
24	USA	70.0
27	Ireland	69.6
134	India	53.2
191	Sierra Leone	25.9

Source: 'Global Patterns of Healthy Life Expectancy', The Lancet, Vol. 357, pages 1685–91 (1999). Reprinted with permission from Elsevier.

We can't all emigrate to Japan or Australia, so how can we increase our life expectancy? Even small changes in diet and lifestyle can bring great health benefits, so will you take up the challenge? That's all you need to do to make this book work for you.

Chapter 2
Diet and lifestyle: the risks and rewards

At first it might seem hard to believe, but it is true:
one diet will help prevent the global epidemic of chronic
disease, and in many cases it may also treat it.

Amazingly, the same pattern of eating can be applied to any ethnic food or cuisine. All right – maybe not the Inuit diet, which consists mainly of seal and fish, and the Masai bushmen's diet, which comprises only meat, milk and blood from their cattle. But the foods preferred by virtually all other cultures can be eaten in the right proportions to make their diet healthy. Simply apply the nutritional guidelines outlined in the latest World Health Organisation (WHO) report on diet and physical activity (summarised in this book on page 160) to eat and enjoy a perfectly balanced diet containing the correct percentage of calories as carbohydrates, protein, dairy food and so on.

The principal recommendations of the report are:

- At least 55 per cent of your daily calories should come from carbohydrates (mainly complex), of which less than 10 per cent should be added sugars.
- Fat should provide no more than 30 per cent of your daily calories, and no more than 10 per cent of this amount should be saturated.
- Protein should provide 10–15 per cent of calories.
- Daily salt consumption should be less than 5 g/1 tsp.
- Eat at least five portions of fruit and vegetables a day.
- Eat 25 g/1 oz of fibre a day.

While these recommendations have been known for a while, the report makes an additional emphasis on the need for 30 minutes to one hour a day of moderate to vigorous physical activity to maintain a healthy body weight.

But we eat food, not nutrients, you might well say. How does that information translate into real food, and how much can you put on your plate if you want to control weight and prevent chronic disease? We'll come to that in Chapter 5, but first it's important to look at some of the scientific evidence behind the healthier food choices and understand how being more physically active can optimise the dietary changes you make.

WEIGHING UP THE EVIDENCE

The proof that you will benefit from eating a healthier diet is mounting, as documented in the WHO report, which rates the evidence on three levels – convincing, probable and possible. More speculative ideas that may or may not increase or decrease the risk are categorised under the heading 'perhaps'.

The scientific evidence is the best currently available from the world's leading independent medical experts and it clearly indicates that healthy eating and a healthy lifestyle can reduce your risk of long-term chronic conditions, such as heart disease, obesity, type 2 diabetes and certain cancers, that threaten us today.

Inevitably, some foods, or substances found in those foods, are more beneficial in lowering the risk of certain diseases than others. For example, a fibre-rich diet helps reduce the risk of all the health problems discussed so far, but it is particularly important in protecting against colon cancer, heart disease and type 2 diabetes. On the other hand, a lower fat diet, especially one low in saturated fat, is protective against lots of diseases, but helps particularly with heart disease and type 2 diabetes.

WHERE DOES THE EVIDENCE COME FROM?

The evidence draws on epidemiological studies that, in this case, look at the diet or physical activity of large numbers of people and then track any association between their diet or exercise levels and how often a specific disease occurs. Other evidence comes from trials that randomly give people different diets or exercise regimes to follow, often over many years, and then compares them with people who did not do anything or did something different. In some cases, laboratory evidence has also supported what has been seen to happen in humans, or come up with explanations for the biological mechanisms that underlie the health problems. These studies also help to explain why one type of nutrient is more beneficial than another.

In addition, the evidence shows that healthy eating will bring you the most benefit if you combine it with being active. Without enough physical activity you won't be able to maintain a healthy body weight, especially if you have a job where you are sitting down all day. How active do you need to be? The report recommends one hour of moderate to vigorous activity each day. If you find that too daunting, there are great benefits to be had from 30 minutes a day (or on most days). Make one hour your long-term goal.

STOP DISEASE BEFORE IT STARTS

The following sections of this chapter deal with the chronic diseases that arise from an unhealthy diet and lifestyle. The first of these is excess weight, which is associated with many other of the diet-related, long-term diseases examined in the WHO report, including cardio-vascular (heart) disease, stroke and high blood pressure, several forms of cancer, type 2 diabetes, osteoporosis and dental disease. As you will see, a diet low in saturated fats, sugars and salt and high in vegetables and fruits, together with regular physical activity, can have a major impact on preventing death and disease.

If you think this does not apply to you, think again. Chronic disease is not someone else's problem – the reality is that it is yours.

Excess weight and obesity

The number of obese people in the UK has tripled over the last 20 years so that one in five adults is now obese – that's 21 per cent of women and 17 per cent of men – and more than half the population is overweight. Worryingly, there is no sign of the trend stopping. Obesity (sometimes referred to as clinical obesity) is defined as having a BMI (body mass index) of 30, while a BMI of 40 is classified as morbid obesity because it poses a serious threat to life. Obesity shortens life expectancy by an average of nine years, and in the UK alone 18 million sick days were attributed to it in 1998 – little wonder when you know that being overweight increases the risk of many long-term health problems, including heart disease, type 2 diabetes, high cholesterol levels, some cancers, high blood pressure and osteo-arthritis.

The chart below shows you at a glance the dietary and lifestyle factors that work for or against the problem of excess weight.

YOUR IDEAL WEIGHT/SIZE

The current thinking is that body mass index (BMI), a calculation based on height and weight, is a better indicator of health than weight alone. Use the steps overleaf to calculate your BMI and find out if you are within the healthy ranges.

GUARD AGAINST OBESITY AND WEIGHT PROBLEMS

Evidence	Decreases risk	Increases risk
Convincing	• Regular physical activity. • High-fibre diet from starchy foods rich in non-starchy polysaccharides (see page 172).	• Too many high-calorie foods. • Sedentary lifestyle.
Probable	• Starting good eating habits from an early age.	• High intake of sugar-sweetened soft drinks.
Possible	• Eating more low glycaemic index foods, which help control hunger and weight gain (see page 169).	• Large portion sizes. • Eating a lot of food prepared outside the home. • Anorexia or bulimia.
Perhaps	• Eating smaller portions more frequently, e.g. six snack meals a day rather than the three-meals-a-day 'norm', but only if the meals are part of a lower fat diet and not additional calories.	• Alcohol might increase weight problems and make abdominal fat more likely; some research suggests it's the snack foods and after-pub take-aways associated with drinking that lead to weight gain. As alcohol increases appetite, there's a tendency to eat more at meals where it is present.

How to calculate your BMI

1. Measure your height in metres and multiply the figure by itself, e.g. 1.6 x 1.6 = 2.56

2. Weigh yourself in kilograms, e.g. 10 stone = 64 kg

3. Divide your weight by the result of step 1, i.e. 64 ÷ 2.56 = 25

Now check your result against the table below.

Less than 18.5	Underweight
18.5–25	Normal range
25+	Overweight
25–29	Pre-obese
30–34	Obese
35–39	Very obese
40+	Extremely obese

Source: 'Diet, Nutrition and the Prevention of Chronic Disease', WHO (2003)

WHY YOUR BMI MATTERS

In the UK half of all adults are overweight, and one in five is obese, with a BMI of 30 or more. The country's average BMI is 26.5 for men and 26.4 for women.

Apart from age, BMI is the most potent predictor for diabetes. Even a score of 25 poses a significantly higher risk than a score of 22, but at more than 30 the risks are enormous – and that includes children too.

IS YOUR BMI HEALTHY?

If your BMI falls within the ideal range, that's great, but it is still important to make sure you stay that way by eating a well-balanced, nutritious diet and taking enough exercise. Even if you are the 'right' weight, you still need to eat nutrient-rich foods to keep your body healthy on the inside and help you to look good and feel even better.

People who stay the same weight throughout middle age live longer and are generally healthier than those who gain weight, and the bonus of this is that they can enjoy their longevity more fully. To enjoy the same benefit, you should aim to weigh the same at 60 (and older) as you did at 30, or certainly not gain more than 5 kg/11 lb during your adult life. Remember, weight gain is associated with a shortened life expectancy up to the age of 75.

SURPRISED BY YOUR BMI?

The BMI chart is a guide – it's not infallible. For example, stocky or muscular people, and children and adolescents during growth spurts, might have BMIs that suggest they're overweight when they're not. Even athletes can have high BMIs because of their dense muscle tissue. If you're disappointed with your BMI, appraise yourself honestly, or ask the opinion of someone you trust. It's true that some people have larger, heavier builds than others, and if you are one of them, it would be a mistake to try to lose weight unnecessarily.

Some experts are concerned that an optimum BMI range of 21–23 is too difficult for many people to achieve, and might tempt them into crash dieting. If you feel the need to lose weight, avoid diets of less than 800 calories per day: they are a risk to health and do nothing to establish healthier eating habits. The diets in this book aim to help you achieve long-term permanent weight correction based on intakes of 1200 calories for women and 1700 for men (see Chapter 5). However, if these levels prove too high for you, they can be reduced, but by no more than 200 calories per day.

Note that the BMI chart opposite is based on Caucasian people, so it cannot be applied to other ethnic groups, such as Polynesians, who have larger body frames, or the Chinese, who have a smaller build. As yet, there is no consensus on what various ethnic BMIs should be. The WHO has suggested a normal range of 18.5–23 for Asians because many Asian countries clearly suffer obesity-related diseases at a lower BMI than Caucasians. Similarly, Australian Aborigines might also need a lower obesity cut-off point (possibly 22) to help prevent the epidemic of glucose intolerance and type 2 diabetes in that population. To date there has been no research specifically on Afro-Caribbeans, but the normal range should account for most individuals. Another drawback of the BMI chart is that its calculations make no allowance for the distribution of fat, which is important in the assessment of risk. Large hips, for example, pose less of a health threat than a 'spare tyre'. In addition, it tells you nothing about the percentage of fat to muscle in your body, which is also very important (see pages 89–90).

IDEAL WEIGHT AND BMI

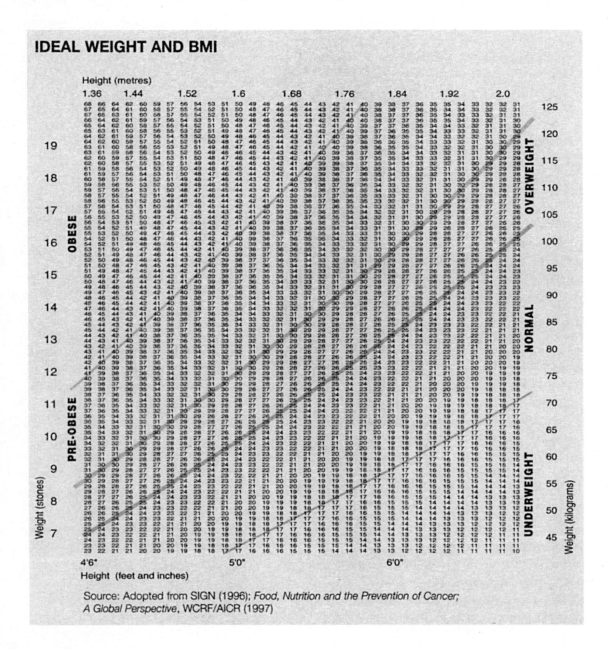

Source: Adopted from SIGN (1996); *Food, Nutrition and the Prevention of Cancer; A Global Perspective*, WCRF/AICR (1997)

Finally, if you are at the top end of the normal range, or perhaps outside it, but are physically fit, then you probably have no excess risk of chronic diseases such as high blood pressure, heart disease and stroke.

APPLES AND PEARS

We each have an in-built genetic pre-disposition to a particular body shape. In women, excess fat tends to be deposited around the upper arms, breasts and hips, resulting in a pear shape, or around the abdomen, resulting in an apple shape. The same is true for men, although they are more likely to have abdominal fat.

Some health risks are associated with extra fat deposits on particular parts of the body. For example, if apple-shaped people become overweight, they are at greater risk of heart disease and type 2 diabetes than pear-shaped individuals. To find out whether you are an apple or a pear, do the following:

- Measure your waist and hips in centimetres.
- Divide the waist measurement by the hip measurement to get your waist–hip ratio, e.g. 86 ÷ 102 = 0.85.

Male pears should have a ratio of less than 0.95 cm, and female pears less than 0.87 cm. Ratios higher than that mean you're an apple.

With abdominal obesity becoming increasingly common, scientists claim that bulging waistlines mark a fundamental change in the

shape and size of humans, an occurrence last seen about 200 years ago when Europeans enjoyed a height gain of about 30 cm/12 in. However, the current worldwide change in shape is more likely to be a mark of disease than improved health.

WAIST SIZE MATTERS TOO

A tape measure can give you another useful indicator of health: men and women who have waist measurements of more than 94 cm/37½ in or 80 cm/32 in respectively are probably overweight and far more likely to develop diabetes. The risks to health increase substantially if the waist measurements are more than 102 cm/41 in or 88 cm/35 in respectively, as at this level men and women are almost certain to be insulin resistant (see page 33) and therefore have problems regulating blood-sugar levels. Of course, waists do thicken with age, a phenomenon often referred to as 'middle-age spread'. However, if you have a spare tyre at any age, act now. Use the information in this book to lose weight and get yourself on track to a healthier future.

YOUR WEIGHT LOSS GOAL

We all know that changing eating patterns and becoming more active are important steps to losing weight and maintaining weight loss. The difficulty for most of us trying to achieve these goals is staying motivated. The best way to do this is to set yourself reasonable and realistic goals. Initially, you should not aim to lose more than 10 per cent of your current body weight (5 per cent is fine), and to do so at a rate of 0.5–1 kg/1–2 lb per week. (For other motivational tips, see page 102.) The best preventive course of action is not to gain weight during adult life, but most of us do – at least 0.5 kg/1 lb a year – and more will be retained by women if weight gained during pregnancy is not lost afterwards. For many people the most realistic goal is to keep weight gain during adult life to a minimum. And if you are starting out in adult life as an overweight teenager, aim not to gain any more excess weight. (For more specific advice on losing and controlling weight, see the exercise ideas in Chapter 4 and the diet and eating plans in Chapter 5.)

Heart disease, stroke and high blood pressure

The main cause of coronary heart disease is atherosclerosis (narrowing and hardening of the arteries), caused by the build-up of fat deposits, such as cholesterol and plaque, on the walls of the arteries. Plaque blocks nutrient delivery to the artery walls, so they harden, which may lead to high blood pressure, a further risk. At the same time, the blood in the narrowed arteries becomes more likely to clot and may block the blood supply to the heart, causing a heart attack or, if it happens in the brain, a stroke.

Unbalanced diets, being overweight and not being active enough all contribute to heart disease, which currently causes an average of nine years' disability in later life, estimated to increase to 14 years by 2020 if bad habits remain unchanged. Insufficient intake of fruit and vegetables, wholegrain cereals, fish or other sources of omega-3 and omega-6 fats, alongside too high an intake of saturated fat and salt, a sedentary lifestyle and smoking specifically increase the risk of heart disease, stroke and high blood pressure. Although you might not yet have any visible or palpable symptoms of heart disease, it is worth making diet and lifestyle changes now because heart disease happens silently over a long period of time.

The chart on page 23 shows you at a glance the dietary and lifestyle factors that work for or

GUARD AGAINST HEART DISEASE, STROKE AND HIGH BLOOD PRESSURE

Evidence	Decreases risk	Increases risk
Convincing	• Maintaining a healthy BMI or body weight (see page 20). • Eating at least five varied portions a day of fruit and vegetables. • 1–2 servings per week of oily fish, or fish oils equivalent to 200 mg of EPA and DHA (see page 73). • Polyunsaturates, such as omega-6 linoleic acid, found in sunflower oil and spreads. • Potassium to lower blood pressure, from daily consumption of fruit and vegetables. • Regular physical activity. • Low to moderate alcohol intake may protect against heart disease, particularly among older women, but doctors don't actually 'recommend' it.	• Being overweight. • Saturated fats and trans fats found in fatty meat, high-fat dairy products and processed foods. • Too much salt is linked to high blood pressure (see page 26). Don't have more than 5 g/1 tsp a day, including that in processed food, ready-made meals and what you add at the table. • Sedentary lifestyle. • High alcohol intake, a specific risk for stroke. Moderate alcohol intake of around three units a day can raise blood pressure.
Probable	• Polyunsaturates, such as omega-3 linolenic acid, found in rapeseed oil, walnuts and some green leafy vegetables. • Monounsaturated oleic acid, found in olive oil. • Non-starchy polysaccharides (NSPs), the collective name for different types of fibre found in whole grains, pulses and certain fruits and vegetables, which lower cholesterol. • Nuts (unsalted). • Folate (found in green leafy vegetables and fortified foods, such as breakfast cereal). • Plant sterols and stanols added to some spreads and foods.	• Too much dietary cholesterol, although saturated fat is more important. • Unfiltered boiled coffee (made on the hob).
Possible	• Flavonoids (antioxidants found in fruit, vegetables, tea and red wine). • Soya products, such as soya protein, lower cholesterol.	• Beta-carotene supplements, shown in trials to make lung cancer more rather than less likely. • Poor nutrition in the womb.
Perhaps	• Minerals: calcium and magnesium, to facilitate electrical messages from the heart and to control blood pressure. • Vitamin C, to protect the heart and build strong blood vessels against stroke.	• Too much refined carbohydrate and sugary food may raise blood fats and lower beneficial cholesterol.

Note: Dietary reference tables that show the amount of each vitamin and mineral you need on a daily basis can be found in Appendix 2 (see page 162), together with easy ways to eat the right amount of food to achieve the recommended intake.

WHOLE GRAINS ARE GOOD FOR YOU

Some experts estimate that three portions of wholegrain cereals a day could help prevent up to a third of heart disease, type 2 diabetes and diet-related cancers of the colon, stomach, mouth and gall bladder. Only 15 per cent of people eat that amount, and many don't even know what whole grains are.

For the uninitiated, whole grains are unrefined cereal products that retain all their fibre. These complex carbohydrates or starches are made into all sorts of foods, such as wholemeal breads and unrefined breakfast cereals, or, like brown rice, cooked just as they are. They are also rich in nutrients and antioxidants that prevent free radicals causing cell damage that leads to cancer and heart disease.

Refining whole grains into white flour for bread, pasta, cakes and biscuits removes about 30 per cent of the nutrients they contain. Since we get around 25 per cent of our energy from grains, and 95 per cent of the grains we eat are white and refined, there is a lot of scope for improving the quality of the food we eat. That's why we should ensure that at least three of the recommended 6–11 daily portions of starchy foods are whole grain.

against the development of heart disease, stroke and high blood pressure.

WHY IS BLOOD PRESSURE IMPORTANT?

Raised blood pressure is a major cause of stroke and heart failure and a significant risk in coronary heart disease, but it can be improved through diet and being more active.

The pumping action of the heart pushes blood around the body, and as the blood circulates, it exerts pressure on the walls of the arteries. The blood pressure is highest when the heart is contracting (systolic pressure), which is represented by the higher figure in a reading. The pressure is lowest between heartbeats (systolic pressure) and is represented by the lower figure in a reading (the height a column of mercury [Hg] reaches from the pressure exerted).

If you have a blood pressure reading that is consistently more than 140/90 mm Hg, you have high blood pressure, which increases your risk of heart problems and stroke. In people aged up to 50 both diastolic blood pressure and systolic blood pressure are independently associated with the risk of heart disease and stroke. At age 50 the systolic (higher) number is far more important then the diastolic (lower) number in predicting the risk of coronary heart disease, heart failure and other related deaths. At age 60 an increasing systolic blood pressure and a lower diastolic reading indicate a higher risk.

The latest recommendation from the US National Heart, Lung and Blood Institute, endorsed by the American Heart Association,

FATS GOOD AND BAD

Although many chronic health problems are a direct result of eating too much saturated fat, we need to eat certain fats that the body cannot make for itself.

Polyunsaturated fats (PUFAs) are found in fish and in plant foods, such as vegetable oils. They are effective at raising levels of beneficial cholesterol and lowering levels of harmful cholesterol (see below). We need about 20 g/¾ oz, and no more than 30 g/1¼ oz of unsaturated fats each day in order to raise levels of beneficial cholesterol and lower levels of harmful cholesterol to help prevent heart disease.

Essential fatty acids (EFAs) are types of polyunsaturated fats that improve blood cholesterol levels and help prevent blood clots. We need at least 4 g a day of omega-6, from linoleic acid, found in sunflower, soya, corn and safflower oils, and 1–2 g of omega-3, from alpha-linoleic acid, found in soya, walnut and linseed oils. Of the two forms of omega-3 – eicosapentaenoic acid (EPA) and docosahexaenoic acid (DHA) – the latter is the most important. Official guidelines from the Food Standards Agency say we need 0.2 g a day, but in the UK we eat only half that amount. The recommendation is that we eat oily fish, such as mackerel, salmon or herring, at least twice a week to ensure a healthy intake of these essential fatty acids.

Monounsaturated fats are good because they reduce levels of harmful cholesterol and increase levels of beneficial cholesterol, although not as effectively as polyunsaturated fats. The best-known monounsaturate is probably olive oil, but monounsaturated fats are also found in rapeseed oil and nuts, especially walnuts. If you need to make up your daily fat allowance, you can do so by including a small amount of monounsaturates.

Saturated fats can be easily distinguished because they are usually solid at room temperature. They include lard, butter, ghee, block margarine and cooking fats. Saturated fats are found mainly in animal products, such as meat, cheese and milk, and in pastries, biscuits and deep-fried food that have been made using butter or vegetable fats high in saturates. An excess of saturates in the diet leads to raised levels of harmful cholesterol in the blood. This can be deposited in the arteries, increasing the risk of heart disease and stroke.

Trans fatty acids start out as unsaturated fats, but the food industry's practice of adding hydrogen to stabilise and harden liquid vegetable oils for cooking purposes and to increase shelf life turns them into trans fats.
   The problem with eating trans fats is that they raise cholesterol levels even more than saturated fats, and increase the risk of heart attack. Responsible food manufacturers try to reduce trans fats, and declare the trans fats content on the ingredients label.

Triglycerides make up most of the fat in the body, and are at their highest level in the bloodstream immediately after a meal. Increasingly, triglycerides are being seen as an independent risk factor for coronary heart disease: the higher the level, the greater the risk. Triglycerides can be reduced in part by eating the right kind of fat, omega-3 in particular.

Cholesterol is a fat that is made by the body because it is essential for building cells, but we also get it from food, particularly dairy products and meat. High-density lipoprotein (HDL) is a beneficial form of cholesterol that seems to protect the arteries from clogging up; low-density lipoprotein (LDL) and very low-density lipoprotein (VLDL) on the other hand are harmful types of cholesterol because they clog up the arteries and contribute to heart disease. For further information about cholesterol, see page 27.

is that everyone with a blood pressure reading higher than 120/80 should be treated for high blood pressure. They advocate bringing blood pressure below 120/80, and ideally down to 115/75. This is in line with WHO goals.

In the USA people with systolic pressure of 120–139 are being termed 'prehypertensive', and the recommendation is that they 'require health-promoting lifestyle modifications to prevent CVD (heart disease and stroke)'. In other words they need to follow the diet and lifestyle advice in *Eat for Life* to prevent chronic disease.

For most people high blood pressure (also known as hypertension) cannot be attributed to any specific cause. However, you are more likely to suffer from it if you are overweight, eat too much salt, too few fruits and vegetables, take little exercise and drink too much alcohol. Blood pressure is very variable, going up when you are angry or stressed (before public speaking, for example), and going down when you are relaxed or asleep. This is why blood pressure may have to be taken several times to get an accurate reading.

HOW CAN DIET HELP YOUR BLOOD PRESSURE?

There is one very simple step you can take to help reduce high blood pressure: cut down your salt intake.

The recommendation is that everyone, not just people with high blood pressure, should cut their salt intake from the current amount of 9–12 g a day (two teaspoonfuls) to no more than 5 g a day (one teaspoonful). If you can reduce the amount even more, it will probably lower your blood pressure even further.

The actual adult requirement for sodium (as 'salt' is listed on ingredients labels) is 1600 mg (1.6 g) a day. But note that sodium is not the same thing as salt (sodium chloride). You need to multiply sodium by 2.5 for its equivalent in salt, which makes the daily requirement 4 g. This is enough for just about every adult, unless you are an Olympic athlete or working in extreme temperature conditions. (Babies, by the way, should not have any added salt.)

Sodium is found in grains, fruits and vegetables, so you don't actually need to add any salt to your food to get adequate amounts. Adding salt is simply a habit that, with a bit of practice, you can easily give up (see below).

HOW TO REDUCE THE AMOUNT OF SALT YOU EAT

Your taste buds get used to the large amount of salt in processed foods and to the amount you add during cooking and at the table. When you stop using salt and reduce salty processed foods, your taste buds will take about three weeks to adapt. If you stop immediately, you will find that food tastes bland, but if you cut down gradually, your taste buds will adjust and you will eventually find that food with added salt masks the real flavour and tastes too salty.

Only about a quarter or less of our salt intake comes from salt that we add during cooking or at the table. The rest is hidden in processed foods, such as bread, cooked meats, high

CHOLESTEROL – FRIEND OR FOE?

Cholesterol has become closely associated in people's minds with meat and dairy products, and there is some justification for this. These foods do contain cholesterol and they do raise blood cholesterol levels, but the rise is generally small. Of far greater effect is the total amount of fat in the diet, particularly saturates and trans fats (see page 25). When we eat too much saturated fat, cholesterol builds up on the walls of the arteries, eventually narrowing them so that a blood clot is more likely to get stuck and cause a heart attack. A high-fat diet, especially one high in saturates, combined with lack of physical exercise and being overweight, is the most common cause of high blood cholesterol in the UK.

As the body makes its own supplies of cholesterol, there is no need to eat any food containing it, although it is hard to avoid in the typical Western diet. The WHO report therefore advises limiting intake to 300 milligramms (mg) a day to keep blood cholesterol within safe bounds. The following examples show how easy it is to eat too much cholesterol.

- 1 medium egg – 200 mg
- 1 portion breaded scampi – 187 mg
- 1 portion of beef mince – 88 mg
- 1 lean pork steak – 65 mg
- 1 matchbox-size piece of Cheddar – 45 mg
- 1 fried chicken wing – 45 mg
- 1 portion shelled prawns – 30 mg
- 1 tbsp cream – 15 mg
- 1 biscuit – 12 mg

If you choose a low saturated fat diet with a moderate intake of meat and fish, you can afford the occasional cholesterol indulgence. Even eggs can be eaten 4–6 times a week in a low-fat diet. Eggs have the advantage over other dairy products and meat in that they do not provide saturated fat.

In the UK the average blood cholesterol for men and women in the 35–65 age range is 6.1–6.2 millimoles per litre (mmol/l), with even higher levels in those aged over 65. These figures are above the UK recommendation of 5.0 mmol/l. Suffice to say, there's a lot of room for improvement.

sodium breakfast cereals, baked beans, crisps and canned soup. For a healthier diet, try to eat more fresh foods.

The famous Dietary Approaches to Stop Hypertension (DASH) trial showed that reducing salt as part of a sensible low-fat diet that includes plenty of fruit and vegetables could reduce blood pressure. For more about the DASH diet, see page 44.

Low sodium products and salt substitutes may be helpful, but ultimately they do not help you to change your taste for salty food. Most salt substitutes mix ordinary salt with potassium chloride and/or magnesium sulphate, so they're not free from sodium and they still taste salty. It is much better to read the label and choose products that contain less salt or sodium than comparable foods in the range. Also add less salt when cooking and at the table.

READ THE LABEL

In the UK nutrition labelling is voluntary unless a nutrition claim (e.g. 'low-fat' or 'high in fibre') is made. However, most food manufacturers now provide the information because customers want it. Nutrition labels therefore appear on most pre-packed foods. You can use this information to your advantage.

Read the label and try to choose products that contain 0.3 g or less of sodium per 100 g of the food. As a guide, 0.5 g of sodium per 100 g (the equivalent of 1.25 g of salt) is a lot, and you might be surprised to find this amount in such items as breakfast cereals and bread. You don't need to avoid these items – in fact, bread and certain cereals are very nutritious and should not be avoided – but you need to be aware of how your salt intake mounts up and choose healthier options.

Cornflakes and some well-known brands of breakfast cereal contain the same concentration of salt as Atlantic sea water – 1 g of sodium per 100g. Would you drink sea water for breakfast?

ALCOHOL AND HEART DISEASE

Perhaps disappointingly, the benefit of alcohol (particularly red wine) to the heart has been overstated. But even if it does offer protection, this must be balanced against other evidence that just one alcoholic drink a day increases the lifetime risk of developing breast cancer by 6 per cent.

It is the antioxidant phenol content of red wine that has led to it being hailed as a heart-saver because polyphenols help prevent hardening of the arteries and mop up harmful free radicals, thereby preventing arteries being silted up with cholesterol. Even though low to moderate alcohol intake may help protect some people from heart disease, the best way to get antioxidants is to eat plenty of fruit, vegetables and wholegrain foods. However, it's understandable that most of us would rather unwind after a busy day with a glass of burgundy than a bunch of grapes...

WHAT ARE THE 'SAFE' LIMITS OF DRINKING?

Until 1995 the Department of Health (DoH) said that the 'safe' amounts of alcohol per week were up to 14 units for women and 21 for men. In an attempt to deter drunkenness and binge drinking, they then suggested that two to three drinks should be the limit on any one occasion. This meant that the weekly limits were raised to 21 units for women and 28 for men. (Yes, it's hard to understand how the DoH thought increasing overall drinking could deter drunkenness.)

A unit of alcohol is the equivalent of one small glass of wine (125 ml), half a pint of beer, or a pub measure of spirit. However, wineglasses in most bars now have a capacity of 175 ml. If the wine is 12 per cent alcohol, this bigger measure provides not one unit but nearly two. Similarly, many beers and lagers now contain more alcohol than previously, so a half pint is also likely to be more than one unit.

HOW MANY UNITS?

In order to know how much you drink, you need to understand how many units of alcohol are in each drink. As most labels on alcoholic drinks do not give this information, you have to work it out yourself. This is easy to do.

1. Find the volume and alcohol percentage on the label, e.g. 75 cl and 13%.

2. Multiply those two figures together:
75 x 13 = 975
3. Divide that figure by 100 for centilitres:
975 ÷ 100 = 9.75 units
4. A typical can of lager tends to be 330 ml with an alcohol content of 5 %. Multiply those two figures: 330 x 5 = 1650, then divide by 1000 = 1.6 units

WOMEN BEWARE

In the UK, women's alcohol consumption has become an area of special concern because one in five is drinking more that the recommended 'safe' level. There are several good reasons why women should not aim to match men drink for drink.

- Women's bodies contain twice as much fat, and alcohol can only be diluted in watery body tissues. It therefore stays longer in the female bloodstream.
- Women's livers are more sensitive to alcohol than men's, putting them at greater risk of cirrhosis.
- Women produce lower amounts of the enzyme needed to detoxify alcohol, so it has a greater effect and stays in their system for longer.
- Drinking alcohol during pregnancy is linked to miscarriage and low birth weight. It can also lead to foetal alcohol syndrome, which produces severely disturbed babies.

Try keeping an alcohol diary for two weeks to check your intake. You could be surprised by the result!

If you would like help in controlling your drinking, contact Drinkline, the National Alcohol Helpline, which offers confidential advice and information on all aspects of alcohol. Call free on 0800 917 8282, Mon–Fri, 11 a.m.–7 p.m.

FOLATES – A FORCE FOR GOOD

Recent research on heart disease has been looking at the influence of homocysteine, an amino acid that is a natural by-product of the breakdown of protein. Raised levels of homocysteine seem to damage the endothelial cells that line the arteries, increasing the risk of heart disease. The good news is that high levels of homocysteine can be counteracted with folates, a type of B vitamin found in green leafy vegetables, whole grains, pulses and liver. Added to fortified foods in the form of folic acid, folates work with vitamins B_{12} and B_6 to reduce elevated levels of homocysteine. We would all benefit from eating more foods that contain folates or folic acid. Rich sources include black-eyed beans, broccoli, Brussels sprouts, fortified breakfast cereals, granary bread, green beans, kale, kidneys, liver, spinach, spring greens and yeast extract. Foods with a medium content of folates include baked beans, brown rice, cauliflower, eggs, iceberg lettuce, oranges, parsnips, peas, potatoes and white bread.

Cancer

Huge advances have been made over the last few decades in the treatment of cancer, but it remains a serious threat to health. New figures suggest that it may overtake heart disease as the number one killer of men in the UK.

There are many causes of cancer – some, such as tobacco, well known, others still to be discovered. Currently, diet accounts for about 30 per cent of cancers in the West (20 per cent in developing countries), making it second only to smoking as a preventable cause of cancer.

Teasing out exactly what foods or diets increase the risk of cancer is difficult because most foods and nutrients interact with each other, and combine with genetic factors and other influences, such as physical activity, to alter cell growth and affect cancer risk from person to person. But some links have already been made. For example, diets that contain a lot of fruit and vegetables reduce the risk of some cancers.

After tobacco, the commonest cause of cancer is being overweight or obese. Cancer of the endometrium (lining of the womb) is three times higher among obese women than lean women, while being overweight is known to increase the risk of breast cancer among post-menopausal women, probably by increasing the amount of oestrogen circulating in the body, which could increase hormone-related tumours. But breast cancer is also the second most common cancer in the world, and the commonest cancer among women, so non-dietary risk factors also play a part. These include a family history of the disease, starting periods at an early age, first pregnancy after age 30 or not having children at all, and late menopause. Poor diet and lack of physical activity may also contribute, and alcohol certainly increases the risk for all women; just one drink a day increases the lifetime risk by 6 per cent.

Prostate cancer in men is associated with a Western-style diet containing high levels of protein and animal fats. Some protection against it may be offered by lycopene, an antioxidant in tomatoes.

WOMEN AT RISK

Four out of five British women are putting themselves at greater risk of cancer by failing to take enough exercise. Most exercise less than three times a week for 30 minutes or more, and one in four women never do any exercise at all.

Research shows that regular exercise can reduce the risk of breast cancer and halve the risk of bowel cancer. It may also prevent lung and endometrial cancer, and even help patients to recover from cancer.

According to a Mori poll for Cancer Research UK, lack of time stops nearly 40 per cent of women from exercising more often. For around 20 per cent of them, lack of motivation was the main issue. (For motivational tips, see page 102)

For more about the links between cancer and excess weight, see Chapter 4, which also offers more information about how exercise can control weight and reduce the risks of chronic disease.

Although deaths from cancer are decreasing in the UK, more people are getting the disease. The best defence against diet-related cancers is to have the right body mass index (see page 19), take enough exercise and improve your diet by eating at least five portions of fruit and vegetables a day.

The chart overleaf shows you at a glance the dietary and lifestyle factors that work for or against cancer.

CAN EATING MEAT GIVE YOU CANCER?

Lean red meat, as part of a diet containing lots of vegetables, fruit and wholegrain cereals, is a nutritious food in moderate amounts. Adults in the UK eat on average about 90 g/3½ oz of beef, lamb, pork or processed meat products each day, the equivalent of 8–10 portions a week. Those who eat more – about 150 g/5 oz a day, or 12–14 portions a week – are advised to eat less.

If you like barbecued food, you should be aware that the blackened bits contain two potential carcinogens: polycyclic aromatic hydrocarbons (PAHs) and heterocyclic amines (HAs). In light of this, health experts recommend not eating barbecued meat, poultry or fish too often.

Eating more than moderate amounts of red meat and processed foods made from it, such

GUARD AGAINST CANCER

Evidence	Decreases risk	Increases risk
Convincing	• Regular exercise. Aim for one hour a day, but 30 minutes is better than none. This specifically lowers the risk for cancers of the colon and rectum. • Maintain weight in the BMI range 18.5–25 (see page 18). • Avoid gaining weight (or more than 5 kg/11 lb) during adult life. • Keep your waist measurement below 80 cm/32 in for women, and 94 cm/37½ in for men.	• Being overweight or obese is associated with cancers of the breast, colorectum, endometrium, oesophagus and kidney. • Alcohol can lead to cancers of the mouth, throat, oesophagus, breast and liver. Avoid alcohol, or drink no more than two units per day, if your main concern is breast cancer. • Moulds, such as aflatoxin (found on nuts and grains), may contribute to liver cancer.
Probable	• Eating at least five varied portions (not less than 400 g/14 oz) of fruit and vegetables a day. Berries and green leafy vegetables seem beneficial against cancers of the mouth, oesophagus, stomach and colorectum. • Physical activity may reduce the risk of breast cancer.	• Eating more than 60 g/2¼ oz per day of preserved meat (sausages, salami, bacon, ham) may increase the risk of colorectal cancer. • Salted preserved foods pose a risk of stomach cancer. • Very hot drinks and food (temperature, not spice), may cause cancers of the mouth, throat and oesophagus.
Possible/Perhaps	• Eating enough high-fibre starchy foods, such as vegetables and fruit, and wholegrain bread, pasta, rice and pulses to bulk food and reduce absorption of carcinogens. Fibre is also fermented in the gut to produce butyrate, which may protect against colorectal cancer. • Regularly eating fish for omega-3 fats. • Nutrients found in food, e.g. carotenoids (orange pigments), vitamins B_2, B_6, folate, B_{12}, vitamins C, D and E. • Minerals, e.g. calcium, zinc, selenium. • Phyto (plant) chemicals, e.g. allium compounds in onions and garlic, isoflavonoids in soya, lignans in whole grains and pulses, oestrogenic effects from cruciferous vegetables, which inhibit enzymes and other processes that allow cancer cells to grow, flavonoids in fruit, and antioxidants in vegetables and red wine.	• Animal fats (from meat and dairy produce). • Amines and hydrocarbons (found in the blackened bits of barbecued or charred meat). • Nitrosamines, carcinogens converted in the colon from nitrites found in smoked, salted and some processed meat products.

Note: Dietary reference tables that show the amount of each vitamin and mineral you need on a daily basis can be found in Appendix 2 (see page 162), together with easy ways to eat the right amount of food to achieve the recommended intake.

as sausages, pies and pâtés, probably increases the risk of cancers of the colon and rectum. It may also increase the risk of breast cancer for women and prostate cancer for men. Meat fat is mainly saturated (see page 25), which on its own may increase the risk of other cancers.

Game, such as venison and hare, is preferable to other red meats because it is leaner. The same is true of game birds, such as pheasant and grouse. In fact, all free-range, wild and organic meat and poultry generally contains less saturated fat than intensively reared animals.

Diabetes

There are 1.5 million people in the UK with type 2 diabetes, and probably a further million who have the disease but are undiagnosed. Although people don't usually die of diabetes, it puts them at four times the risk of heart disease and stroke.

In type 2 diabetes not enough insulin is produced in the body, or people become resistant to the effect of it, which doctors call 'insulin resistance' or 'impaired glucose tolerance'. Insulin is the hormone needed for carbohydrates (broken down to glucose during digestion) to be taken from the blood into body cells. It also transports amino acids (broken down from protein) to body cells. The body's failure to make enough insulin results in a potentially dangerous build-up of sugar in the blood.

Type 2 diabetes, which is directly related to diet and lifestyle, used to occur around the age of 40. Nowadays, however, poor diet and a sedentary lifestyle mean that it is being diagnosed much sooner – as early as the age of 11.

Type 2 diabetes is usually related to being overweight, particularly among apple shapes, who carry their excess weight mainly around the middle. Lack of physical activity often contributes to the weight problems that lead to diabetes, but a sedentary lifestyle is also a risk factor in its own right.

The chart overleaf shows you at a glance the dietary and lifestyle factors that work for or against the disease.

WHAT'S THE TREATMENT FOR TYPE 2 DIABETES?
Correcting the balance of foods in the diet and increasing the level of physical activity can reverse the early symptoms of type 2 diabetes, or prevent them occurring if they haven't yet appeared.

The first step is to lose weight, if necessary, then replace most of the saturated fats in your diet with unsaturated fats (see page 25), and increase the proportion of starchy food that is both rich in fibre and has a low glycaemic index (see page 168).

The good news is that taking more exercise and reducing weight can cure – and definitely prevent – type 2 diabetes.

GUARD AGAINST TYPE 2 DIABETES

Evidence	Decreases risk	Increases risk
Convincing	• Losing weight if overweight or obese (see page 19). • Avoiding excessive adult weight gain. • Taking one hour of vigorous activity every day is the ideal, but 30 minutes may be a more achievable target. Try to ensure regular, daily activity.	• Being overweight or obese (see page 19). • Abdominal obesity (spare tyre) round the middle. • Sedentary lifestyle. • Family history of diabetes, including gestational diabetes (during pregnancy) on the maternal side.
Probable	• Eating more wholegrain or complex carbohydrate foods that are high in fibre, e.g. breads and cereals, beans and pulses, vegetables and fruit.	• Too much saturated fat in the diet; it should account for less than 10 per cent of daily calories (see page 160).
Possible	• Getting enough omega-3 fats (see page 25). • Eating more low glycaemic index foods (see page 169).	• Too much fat (of all kinds) in the diet. • Too many trans fats (see page 25).
Perhaps	• Moderate alcohol intake may help control blood sugar in post-menopausal women with diabetes by improving insulin sensitivity, whether the women are overweight or not. • Getting enough vitamin E and other antioxidants helps prevent damage to cells by free radicals. Diabetes leads to raised levels of free radicals, which can damage artery walls and allow cholesterol to build up on them as plaque. Trials giving diabetics 800–1200 iu of vitamin E daily have reduced levels to those of non-diabetics.	• Too much alcohol. Zero or moderate intake may protect against diabetes, so drink within 'safe' guidelines (see page 29).

Note: Dietary reference tables that show the amount of each vitamin and mineral you need on a daily basis can be found in Appendix II (see page 162), together with easy ways to eat the right amount of food to achieve the recommended intake.

EATING WELL WITH DIABETES

A healthy diet for people with diabetes is much the same as for everyone else. However, those with diabetes need advice for their particular case from a diabetes nurse or dietitian, and regular monitoring by their GP.

People who use insulin or other medication to regulate their diabetes should eat regularly, and most need to snack to help control the effects of their medication. The best types of snack are fresh fruit, plain biscuits, wholegrain breads or a glass of milk.

Meals should be based on the right amount of starchy foods for each individual, preferably wholegrain varieties, as these improve sensitivity to insulin. Eat plenty of fruit and vegetables, as well as beans, peas and lentils, but remember that the amount you can eat of most of these foods will need to be controlled. Small portions of lean meat and low-fat milk, yoghurt and cheese will help keep saturated fat intake down, as will keeping deep-fried foods, cakes, pastries, chocolates and other fatty foods for special occasions only. Regular consumption of oily fish is also beneficial.

Small amounts of ordinary sugar are acceptable in high-fibre wholegrain breakfast cereals, yoghurts and low-fat cakes such as wholemeal scones. Special diabetic cakes and confectionery are not necessary – or desirable – because they are often as fatty as standard ones. In fact, the Food Standards Agency and the UK's leading diabetes charity have condemned such products as overpriced and of no real benefit.

Avoid added sugar in tea and coffee, and drink plenty of water. With soft drinks, choose 'diet' or unsweetened varieties. If you drink alcohol, never do so on an empty stomach as this can accelerate hypoglycaemia (low blood-sugar levels, caused by sugar being cleared too quickly from the bloodstream). This can lead to dizziness, weakness and eventually collapse if sugar or glucose, for such emergencies, is not taken.

LIVING WITH DIABETES

Alongside a normal, healthy balanced diet, people with diabetes should take regular exercise because it helps control weight and improves the body's sensitivity to insulin.

It is essential to check with your doctor, diabetic nurse or dietitian about how to increase your activity level safely in order to avoid any over-strenuous exercise or sudden changes that might unbalance insulin levels. And if you take insulin or tablets for diabetes, it is essential to seek professional help in adjusting food and medication before and after exercise to avoid potentially harmful highs and lows in blood sugar.

TYPE 1 DIABETES

Unlike type 2 diabetes, type 1 diabetes is much rarer and not directly related to diet and lifestyle. It often occurs early in life, when the insulin-producing cells in the pancreas are destroyed by a dysfunction of the auto-immune system. This leads to hyperglycaemia (raised levels of blood sugar) and requires regular injections of insulin to control blood-sugar levels. Sometimes type 2 diabetes can progress to the point where the body fails to produce insulin, in which case medication may be needed.

For both types of diabetes, consult your doctor about diet and lifestyle.

METABOLIC SYNDROME

First recognised more than 20 years ago, metabolic syndrome (also known as syndrome X) describes a group of symptoms that may or may not indicate a pre-diabetic state. More definite is that it certainly puts people at higher risk of heart disease.

Currently fashionable, the syndrome has been wrongly used to justify potentially unhealthy low-carbohydrate diets and high-protein or high-fat diets, which consist mainly of meat and dairy foods. Some proponents wrongly claim that insulin resistance causes obesity. In fact, the reverse is true: weight gain causes insulin resistance.

US research has pinpointed several signs that indicate if people are suffering from metabolic syndrome:
• Abdominal obesity greater than 102 cm/41 in (men) and 88 cm/35 in (women).
• Elevated levels of triglycerides greater than or equal to 1.15 mmol/l.
• Low HDL cholesterol levels of less than 1.4 mmol/l (men) and 1.03 mmol/l (women).
• Elevated blood pressure greater than or equal to 130/85 mm Hg.
• Fasting level of blood glucose greater than 6.11 mmol/l.

All these symptoms indicate a higher risk of heart disease. It is also recognised that insulin resistance is a contributory factor to metabolic syndrome.

The best way to deal with this plethora of symptoms is lifestyle change – eating a healthy diet, being physically active and, if necessary, losing weight and taking medication for the high blood pressure. Regular exercise and weight control are also the best ways to reduce the risk of diabetes and to control blood-sugar levels.

In support of this advice, three major diabetes prevention studies in Finland, the USA and the Netherlands show that gradually losing 3–4 kg/7–9 lb in weight more than halves the risk of type 2 diabetes for people showing signs of pre-diabetes or metabolic syndrome. Such weight loss can prevent or delay the age at which type 2 diabetes develops.

Neither a low-carbohydrate diet (below 30 per cent of total intake, but often much lower) nor a high-protein diet (above 20 per cent of total calories as protein) or a high fat diet (more than 40 per cent calories as fat) is the answer as none is sensibly balanced. The healthier option is to eat more wholegrain carbohydrates, more pulses, nuts and seeds, more vegetables and fruits, more fish and seafood than meat, and to replace saturated fat with unsaturated.

Osteoporosis

Osteoporosis is a disease in which the bones lose minerals and take on a sponge-like appearance. As they weaken and become increasingly more fragile, bones become more likely to fracture, break or cause pain and postural problems, such as a stooped back. Common fracture sites include the wrist, hip and spine.

Bone loss occurs with age and accelerates in women around and after the menopause. In the UK, osteoporosis is estimated to affect 3 million people aged over 50 – that's one in three women and one in 12 men in the relevant age group. As the proportion of older people in the population continues to increase, it is estimated that hip fractures will increase fourfold by the year 2050.

The chart overleaf shows you at a glance the dietary and lifestyle factors that work for or against the disease.

WHO IS AT RISK?

Hip fracture rates are highest among white post-menopausal women living in temperate climates. Fracture rates are somewhat lower in women from Mediterranean and Asian countries, and lowest in women from Africa. Heavy people have stronger bones than slight people with a low BMI or body weight. Family history also plays a part in increasing or decreasing the risk: for example, if your mother had osteoporosis, your own risk of developing it is greater too.

Medical conditions that require long-term use of steroids or anti-coagulants significantly increase the risk, as do Crohn's disease and other gut-absorption problems, anorexia, over-exercising, early menopause and hysterectomy.

Other factors that can increase the risk include a lifetime of insufficient calcium and other vitamins and minerals, and taking too little load-bearing exercise. These things are especially important before the age of 25 because childhood and adolescence are the time for building up bone density.

People aged 50 and over must ensure they get enough calcium (from dairy foods, or vegetarian sources, such as fortified soya products, nuts, vegetables and bread). They must also get a good intake of vitamin D (from dairy foods and butter or fat spreads, eggs and the action of sunlight on the skin).

THE CALCIUM PARADOX

Strange but true: hip fracture rates are higher in developed countries where calcium intake is greater than in developing countries (or Japan) with a low calcium intake where hip fractures are rare. Why is this?

It seems that a high-protein diet based on animal sources (as in the Western diet) may negate some of the protective benefit of calcium. It's not clear why this is, but it may be due to the effect of animal protein on blood acidity. Breaking down animal protein (meat) generates acid, which the body has to buffer by mobilising calcium (an alkali) from the bones and teeth.

GUARD AGAINST OSTEOPOROSIS

Evidence	Decreases risk	Increases risk
Convincing	• Adequate intake of vitamin D and calcium. • Regular lifetime physical activity, especially load-bearing exercise, e.g. brisk walking or climbing stairs. In later life activities that build muscle and improve coordination and balance are also important. • Healthy body weight or BMI (see pages 18 and 20).	• High alcohol intake. • Low body weight and anorexia. • Sedentary lifestyle. • Low calcium and vitamin D intake.
Possible	• Low salt intake. • Fruit, vegetables and soya products because they contain beneficial phyto-oestrogens (plant hormones), potassium, magnesium and boron, and because they encourage alkalinity in the body (see Alkalising Diet, page 46). • Moderate alcohol intake (no more than two units a day), but this does not mean that you should drink.	• High salt intake. • Diet high in animal protein rather than vegetable protein. • Low protein intake in older people.

Note: Dietary reference tables that show the amount of each vitamin and mineral you need on a daily basis can be found in Appendix 2 (see page 162), together with easy ways to eat the right amount of food to achieve the recommended intake.

Bones and teeth are in a state of flux throughout life, giving up and re-depositing calcium and other minerals, but the process becomes less effective with age. When the body mobilises lots of calcium to buffer an acid diet, it is likely to be lost later in the urine and not put back into bones.

Digesting plant foods, which are rich in potassium, creates an alkaline environment that is conducive to laying down minerals and building new bone cells, a lifelong process. Genetics, lifestyle and geography (minerals imparted to food through the soil and water) also seem to produce different calcium requirements for different peoples. In the Far East and Africa, for example, bone density tends to be lower than in the West, yet the rates of osteoporosis and related bone fractures are lower.

CAN PHYTO-OESTROGENS HELP BONES?

After the menopause the body stops producing oestrogen, the female sex hormone that protects against osteoporosis. This is one of the reasons why oestrogen is given to women in hormone replacement therapy. However, oestrogen is not trouble-free and the amount needed to encourage bone health may increase the risk of breast cancer for some women. This is where phyto (plant) oestrogens come in.

One theory why there might be a low incidence of osteoporosis in Asian women eating a traditional diet is the high intake of soya products rich in plant oestrogens. These oestrogens stimulate bones but not breast tissue, so, in theory, they do not have the potential to increase the risk of breast cancer. Eating more plant foods rich in oestrogens may help prevent osteoporosis, although research on Far Eastern women suggests it is a regular lifetime exposure to soya foods that is of greatest benefit.

Dental disease

While dental disease may seem relatively unimportant – after all, you don't die from it – treating it costs more than heart disease, osteoporosis or diabetes. Over the period 1999–2000 the UK government spent a staggering £2.2 billion on teeth. Of course, everyone wants a nice white smile, but there's more at stake than self-esteem. Dental disease can seriously limit what people eat and therefore contribute to poor nutrition.

The main cause of dental caries (decay) and loss of teeth is diet, principally too much sugar. During the Second World War, when sugar was rationed, dental health was much better than now. More recently, peoples such as the Inuit, the Sudanese and the Ethiopians, who have shifted to eating Western foods and thereby increased their sugar consumption, suffer far more dental caries than previously.

Frequent consumption of sugar, as seen among confectionery workers, also results in a higher than average incidence of dental caries. The worst scenario of all for dental caries is poor diet (low nutrient intake) coupled with a frequent high sugar intake. As might be expected, the children of dentists suffer less tooth decay than others, no doubt because

their dental health is closely monitored and probably because they have restricted access to sugary foods.

The chart overleaf shows you at a glance the dietary and lifestyle factors that work for or against the problem of dental disease.

NATURAL SUGARS

It has been suggested that fruit and starchy foods, such as bread, pasta, rice and potatoes, are as harmful to teeth as added sugars because the natural sugar and starch have the potential to ferment in the mouth and cause decay. In fact, it is mainly refined sugars, such as table sugar, honey, fructose and sucrose that have been extracted from their wholefood environment, that cause problems. As for the fibre component of starch, this is fermented in the gut, with only beneficial effects (see page 75), so starchy foods do not increase the risk of tooth decay in the same way that sugars do.

STEPS TO IMPROVE DENTAL HEALTH

Fluoride is a mineral that binds with tooth enamel to make the teeth stronger and give greater resistance to decay. It also reduces acid production in dental plaque. These benefits are particularly important during childhood, when the teeth are developing.

Alongside a good diet that includes lots of fruit, vegetables and starchy carbohydrates, cleaning the teeth at least twice a day with a fluoride toothpaste and regular flossing (adults only) are the best measures to prevent caries. You certainly don't have to drink fluoridated

GUARD AGAINST DENTAL PROBLEMS

(caries, erosion, enamel defects and gum disease)

Evidence	Decreases risk	Increases risk
Convincing	• Brushing with fluoride toothpaste. • Good oral hygiene. Electric toothbrushes are more effective than manual. Floss once a day. • Absence of plaque. • Vitamin D to prevent enamel defects.	• Eating more than 40 g/1½ oz of free sugars a day, i.e. table sugar and sugars in sweets, cakes and biscuits. • Eating foods containing free sugars, or having a high intake of sugary drinks. • Deficiency of vitamin C can lead to gum disease. • Excessive fluoride can damage enamel development.
Probable	• Hard cheese, particularly if taken at the end of a meal rather than a pudding. • Sugar-free chewing gum, as it promotes saliva flow that helps clean the teeth	
Possible	• Xylitol, an artificial sweetener used in gum and foods. • Drinking milk; the minerals offer protection, and the naturally occurring milk sugar (lactose) does no harm. • Dietary fibre; probably helps to clean teeth and keep gums healthy.	• Under-nutrition; babies and children who are underfed or undernourished are more likely to have tooth decay.
Perhaps	• A diet high in whole fresh fruit may be protective.	• Dried fruits, which contain lots of sugars, may be a risk (like sugar) if eaten too frequently.

Note: Dietary reference tables that show the amount of each vitamin and mineral you need on a daily basis can be found in Appendix 2 (see page 162), together with easy ways to eat the right amount of food to achieve the recommended intake.

water to benefit. In fact, too much fluoride during the early years can cause fluorosis, an unsightly mottling of the teeth, and damage enamel.

THE REWARDS ARE WORTH IT

As you have seen, this chapter shows that one diet truly does 'fit all'. In combination with enough physical activity, it can help you to lose weight and keep in shape so that you need never regain those pounds. Weight control is a powerful enough motivator in itself, but the scientific evidence that healthy eating and exercise can also guard against disease is even more compelling. By adjusting what you eat and your level of activity, you can enjoy the benefits of avoiding or delaying heart disease, certain cancers, diabetes, osteoporosis – and even save on your dental bills.

Chapter 3
Twenty key foods

Food is a major source of pleasure in life, so mealtimes should be enjoyable occasions, providing an opportunity to experiment with the many foods and flavours from around the world.

For a healthy diet you need a wide variety of foods. Eating 20 or more biologically different foods a day will help you to achieve the necessary balance.

Healthy eating does not require you to give up any foods, but you might need to eat less of certain foods to get the right balance in your diet. A healthy diet is one that relies on a wide variety of foods, each contributing their own particular benefits. And while there are certainly some foods that you should eat more of – such as the 20 highlighted in this chapter – you should not lose sight of the overall picture of your diet.

MAJOR FOOD GROUPS

Vegetables and fruits – a huge variety of plant foods, of which all parts – from the root to the growing tips – may be used

Carbohydrates – whole grains, bread, pasta, rice and starchy vegetables, such as potato, cassava, sweet potato and yam

Protein – fish, poultry, meat and game (preferably lean) and vegetarian alternatives, such as tofu and other soya products, pulses and Quorn

Dairy foods – milk, cheese and yoghurt (preferably low-fat)

Fats and oils – vegetable oils (preferably rich in polyunsaturates or monounsaturates, with as little saturated fat as possible)

Principles of a healthy daily diet

The way to achieve a healthy pattern of eating can be summed up in the following three steps:

1. Eat five or more portions of fruit and vegetables.

2. Eat 6–11 portions of starchy carbohydrates. The exact amount depends on how many calories you need, which in turn depends on your age, sex, size and level of physical activity.

3. Reduce the amount of saturated fat you consume, while ensuring you eat a small but vital amount of unsaturated fat (see page 25).

You can see at a glance how to achieve these steps if you look at the diagrams opposite produced by the UK Department of Health and the US Department of Agriculture.

The National Food Guide for the UK, as depicted in the Healthy Eating Plate (opposite top), represents the basic proportions of foods that go to make up a healthy diet. The proposed reworking of the US Food Pyramid (opposite bottom) emphasises that long-term health relies on a foundation of physical activity to keep you fit and maintain your weight in the healthy range. It also emphasises that the quality of food you eat is important. For example, replace saturated fats from meat and dairy products with unsaturated fats from fish, nuts and seeds, and replace refined white sugary carbohydrates with starchy whole grains, such as pulses, potatoes, bread, brown rice and wholemeal pasta.

THE BALANCE OF GOOD HEALTH

The Foods Standards Agency plate model of a healthy diet for the UK.

Reproduced by kind permission of the Food Standards agency

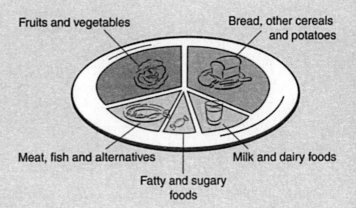

Fruits and vegetables

Bread, other cereals and potatoes

Meat, fish and alternatives

Milk and dairy foods

Fatty and sugary foods

THE HEALTHY EATING PYRAMID

Proposed new US model for healthy eating.

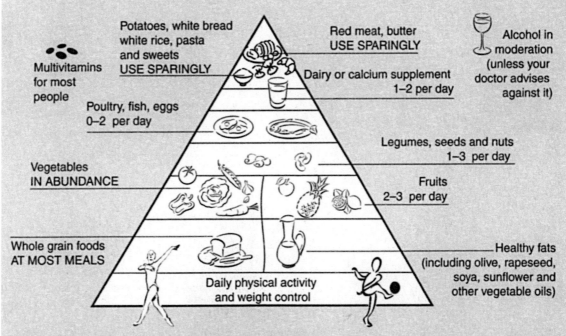

Multivitamins for most people

Potatoes, white bread white rice, pasta and sweets
USE SPARINGLY

Red meat, butter
USE SPARINGLY

Dairy or calcium supplement
1–2 per day

Alcohol in moderation (unless your doctor advises against it)

Poultry, fish, eggs
0–2 per day

Legumes, seeds and nuts
1–3 per day

Vegetables
IN ABUNDANCE

Fruits
2–3 per day

Whole grain foods
AT MOST MEALS

Daily physical activity and weight control

Healthy fats (including olive, rapeseed, soya, sunflower and other vegetable oils)

Reprinted with the permission of Simon & Schuster Publishing Group from *Eat, Drink and Be Healthy: The Harvard Medical School Guide to Healthy Eating* by William C. Willett, MD, copyright © 2001 by President and Fellows of Harvard College

Different ways to healthy eating

Following the guidelines in the healthy eating diagrams will reduce your risk of all the chronic diseases discussed in Chapters 1 and 2, but they do not mean you have to adopt a restrictive diet. Many cultures have interesting and healthy diets that have evolved naturally from the ingredients available locally, and the principles of these can be adapted to improve the balance of the typical Western diet.

Here we look at some of those diets, each of which has different ways of bringing health benefits to your eating pattern.

LOW-SALT DASH DIET

A trial called Dietary Approaches to Stop Hypertension (DASH) gave its name to a diet that reduced the amount of red meat, sweets and sugary soft drinks in order to see if it would lower blood pressure. The results were encouraging, but it was found that the diet worked best when salt intake was lowered too. In fact, it works both to prevent and treat high blood pressure.

To further test the efficacy of the diet, a follow-up trial put the participants on different levels of sodium for 30 days after the main trial. The results were conclusive: the blood pressure of those who ate a high-sodium or medium-sodium diet went back up, but came down when they returned to the low-sodium diet. The principles of the DASH diet (2000 calories a day) are outlined on the right.

DID YOU KNOW?

The most popular sources of carbohydrate – white bread, cakes, biscuits, sugars, syrups, refined cereals and soft drinks – account for half our food intake, but they are the wrong sort. Ideally, choose unrefined, wholegrain carbohydrates, which provide more nutrients.

Daily allowances
- 7–9 portions of starchy foods (bread, cereals, rice, pasta and potatoes, fruit scone, teacake, rice cakes), choosing wholegrain types whenever possible
- 4–5 portions of vegetables
- 4–5 portions of fruit
- 2–3 portions of low-fat dairy foods
- 2 or fewer portions of lean meat, fish or poultry
- 2–3 portions of foods containing unsaturated fat

Weekly allowances
- 4–5 portions of nuts, seeds or beans
- no more than 5 portions of sweet treats

MEDITERRANEAN DIET

Although not particularly low in fat, the Mediterranean diet has a reputation for protecting against cancer and heart disease. This is believed to stem from it containing a healthier balance of common Western foods.
- Olive oil is used in salad dressings and in place of saturated fats for cooking, so the diet has a higher proportion of monounsaturated fat than other Western diets.

- Pulses, such as beans and chickpeas, are eaten regularly.
- Nuts are eaten regularly.
- Bread, as well as other cereals, is eaten regularly.
- Fruit is eaten in higher quantities.
- Vegetables are eaten in larger amounts.
- Meat and meat products are eaten less frequently.
- Milk and dairy products are eaten in moderation.
- Wine is drunk regularly and in moderation with food.

Although olive oil is seen as a key component of a Mediterranean diet and is essential for many of its delicious foods, the same health effect can be achieved by using mainly sunflower oil, a polyunsaturated fat.

HEALTHY VEGETARIAN DIET

Avoiding meat and other animal products does not necessarily make for a healthier diet. In fact, vegetarian diets can be very unhealthy if they contain a lot of refined (white) carbohydrates and high-fat foods because hydrogenated and trans fats from processed vegetable oils are as harmful as saturated fat from animal sources. Refined carbohydrate diets also lack protective plant nutrients and fibre.

The best kind of vegetarian diet is based on the following principles.
- Low consumption of saturated animal fat – only vegans avoid all animal fat, including dairy foods
- Lots of fruit
- Lots of vegetables
- Regular inclusion of nuts

- Regular inclusion of cereals, particularly wholegrain cereals

PRUDENT PLAN OR MODERATE MIXED DIET

One large study of diet and health followed health professionals for eight years and showed that people who ate a 'prudent' Western diet had a lower risk of heart disease and other problems than those who ate an unregulated Western diet, typically high in fatty and sugary foods.

The main principles of the prudent pattern are.
- Lots of fruit
- Lots of vegetables
- Inclusion of pulses, such as beans and lentils
- Inclusion of wholegrain cereals
- Inclusion of fish and poultry
- Not too much of anything – the essence of prudence

HEALTHY JAPANESE DIET

The traditional Japanese diet has had many health claims made for it because the Japanese who eat it have the longest life expectancy and low rates of heart disease.

Typically, it is low in fat and sugar and regularly contains the following foodstuffs.
- Lots of soya, such as tofu and beans
- Seaweeds, rich in the minerals iodine (for thyroid function) and selenium (an anti-oxidant) which are often lacking in a Western diet
- Raw fish, rich in minerals and in omega-3 fats
- Rice, rather than wheat, as the staple starchy food

ALKALISING DIET

Diets high in animal protein have been found more likely to encourage osteoporosis than plant-based diets, and may also influence some diet-related cancers. This is possibly because plant-based foods have an alkalising effect on the blood, which encourages bone remineralisation. A diet rich in animal products and fatty, sugary foods, on the other hand, makes the body more acidic.

An alkalising diet based on the proportions in the Healthy Eating Plate (see page 43) regularly includes:
- Whole grains, such as brown rice and oats, plus potatoes and sweet potatoes
- Vegetables, especially dark green leafy vegetables, all members of the cabbage family, carrots, squash, peppers, onions, peas, avocados, celery, salad leaves, fresh green herbs and root vegetables
- Pulses, including all varieties of beans, lentils, chickpeas and soya products
- Nuts and seeds
- Fish and shellfish
- Poultry and eggs
- Limited amounts of low-fat milk, or soya milk fortified with vitamins and minerals
- Occasional lean red meat, coffee and tea, but mainly water, green tea or herb teas to drink

What do all these healthy diets have in common?
- They are low in saturated fat and the best ones are very low in trans fats.
- They provide a balanced ratio of omega-6 to omega-3 fats from fish and/or plant foods and nuts.
- They provide a higher than average unsaturated fat content.
- They incorporate a wide variety of fruit and vegetables in higher than average amounts.
- They are low in salt.
- They all contain small amounts of protein foods (e.g. meat, fish, eggs and dairy products).

Twenty key foods to eat for life

1. Leaves
2. Root vegetables
3. Vegetable bulbs
4. Stalks and stems
5. Fruiting vegetables
6. Pods and seeds
7. Fruit
8. Whole wheat
9. Other whole grains
10. Breakfast cereal
11. Rice
12. Nuts
13. Pulses
14. Fats and oils
15. Fish
16. Yoghurt and probiotics
17. Milk and cheese
18. Lean red meat and game
19. Poultry
20. Seaweed

The most important contribution to healthy eating is to eat at least five portions of fruit and vegetables a day. Be as colourful and varied in your choice as you can and regularly choose from the different parts of plants – leaves, roots, stalks, seeds, fruit, etc. – because they all make different nutritional contributions to your diet and they each contain different protective chemicals.

1. Leaves

Eat as part of the recommended five or more daily portions of fruit and vegetables.

Green leafy vegetables are wonderfully nutritious. They include cabbage, spinach, broccoli, kale and Brussels sprouts, salad leaves, vine leaves, Swiss chard, lettuce, purslane, rocket, sorrel… and no doubt you can add a few favourites of your own to the list.

Generally, the darker the colour, the higher the nutrient and fibre content. Brassicas (members of the cabbage family) contain glucosinolates and other plant nutrients that may protect against cancer. Lettuce, broccoli, spinach, kale and Chinese leaves, such as pak choi, are also good sources of folates and relatively rich in calcium. In common with Brussels sprouts and cabbage, they also provide vitamin C, while spinach, sprouts and watercress also provide iron.

The fibre content of green leafy vegetables protects against digestive cancers. Some stimulate production of anti-cancer enzymes, while others contain sulphur compounds that kill harmful bacteria.

Salad leaves, which are usually eaten raw, offer

many benefits because their enzyme and nutrient content is not destroyed or diminished by cooking. In general, the darker their colour – whether green, red or purple – the higher their antioxidant content. In fact, one study showed that the maroon-coloured lollo rosso lettuce contained 100 times more antioxidant flavonols than pale green lettuce. Similarly, the darker the leaves, the more vitamins, folic acid and iron they contain.

For greatest vitamin conservation, buy whole lettuce rather than ready-prepared leaves, and tear rather than cut the leaves with a knife.

Easy ways to eat more leaves
Use Leaves in stir-fries. Chinese leaves, cabbage and broccoli are excellent additions to stir-fries, as is chard.

Include a green leafy vegetable with another vegetable of contrasting colour when serving traditional meals consisting of meat or fish with veg.

Eat salads all year round, not just during the summer. Add colour and crunch to them by including extras such as shredded red cabbage, radishes, grated carrots or raw beetroot. Get into the habit of having a side salad to accompany toasted sandwiches, pizza or pasta dishes. To turn salads into more substantial main meals, add protein, such as nuts, beans, poultry or fish, and serve with wholegrain bread or a baked potato.

Give greater texture, colour and flavour to sandwich fillings by adding salad leaves. The same goes for wraps and other flat breads, which can be stuffed even fuller with leaves.

Make dishes look more appetising by adding garnishes, such as watercress, lamb's lettuce or other attractive salad leaves, and don't forget to eat them too.

Use all sorts of leaves to make soups. (Invest in a good cookbook for inspiration.)

Make juices based on vegetables and fruit, adding salad leaves and herbs for extra flavour.

Add the distinctive flavour of herbs, such as coriander, basil, parsley, tarragon, oregano and marjoram, to simple green salads.

Grow your own herbs and salad leaves in the garden or window boxes so that you have a ready supply always to hand. Choose more unusual or expensive varieties, such as rocket, purslane and Good King Henry.

Dress it up
The dressing you eat with salads is a great opportunity to add beneficial fats to the diet. Make salad dressings from extra virgin olive oil or soya, sunflower, safflower and corn oil, all of which are high in unsaturated fats. To ring the changes, try some of the more unusual unsaturated oils, such as walnut, hazelnut and avocado. Let mayonnaise with salad become a thing of the past and you will gain benefits in both flavour and health.

2. Root vegetables
Eat as part of the recommended five or more daily portions of fruit and vegetables.

As their name suggests, root vegetables grow underground. Most of them are rich in fibre and contain a wealth of nutrients that makes them an essential part of a healthy diet.

Root vegetables such as potatoes, yam, sweet potato and taro, the staples of many cultures, are classified as carbohydrates because, unlike other vegetables, they are staple foods eaten mainly for energy rather than their vitamin and mineral content. In the UK potatoes are eaten in such quantity that they make a major contribution to our vitamin C intake, despite not being very rich in that vitamin.

The non-staple root vegetables, such as carrots and sweet potatoes, contain beta-carotene, an antioxidant that gives them their colour and helps to improve night vision. Their carotenoid content also protects the lens of the eye from damage by ultraviolet light and thereby reduces the risk of cataracts. Eating lots of vegetables high in carotenoids (basically anything orange or yellow) is associated with a low risk of lung and respiratory problems. (Carotenoid supplements do not provide the same benefit.)

Beta-carotene also helps the body to absorb iron from grains because it blocks the effect of iron-binding phytochemicals such as phytic acid, found in the bran part of grains. Beetroot contains a different type of carotene that may have other protective effects against carcinogens. Both carrots and sweet potato are also good sources of vitamin C, as are radishes and the unfashionable and under-used swede and turnip. Taro too is an excellent source of vitamin C, and contributes iron, more commonly associated with green vegetables. Unusually for a vegetable, sweet potato is a source of the antioxidant vitamin E.

Another contribution of starchy root vegetables is non-starchy polysaccharides (NSPs), including both insoluble fibre (e.g. cellulose) and soluble fibre (e.g. gums and pectins). The best known benefit of insoluble fibre is the prevention and cure of constipation, but it also speeds up the transit time of waste materials through the gut. As a prebiotic fibre, it is a special 'food' for beneficial gut bacteria.

Most vegetables are good sources of fibre, but be adventurous and try some of the more unusual ones, such as celeriac. Artichokes are a good source of soluble fibre, which is fermented to produce anti-cancer agents and other substances that boost the immune system. Soluble fibre also helps to transport harmful cholesterol from the body, thus fighting heart disease.

Beetroot, yam and all varieties of potato are excellent sources of potassium, which is important for regulating blood pressure.

In the Western diet root vegetables are usually steamed or boiled, but they are endlessly adaptable and can be cooked in a variety of ways. Look at the ideas below and build more root vegetables into your diet.

Easy ways to eat more root vegetables
Serve 2 portions of vegetables (in addition to potatoes, rice, noodles or pasta) at your main meal.

Purée cooked vegetables, such as parsnips and carrots, to make soups.

Make nutritious drinks by juicing your favourite vegetables. For a start, try carrots or beetroot with apple.

Grate raw vegetables, such as carrots and celeriac, and use in salads and sandwiches.

Add grated or finely diced carrot, parsnip and swede to dishes such as shepherd's pie, lasagne, curry and moussaka. Family members who 'don't like vegetables' might not be so reluctant to eat them if they are part of a prepared dish.

Roast vegetables, lightly brushed with olive oil or vegetable oil, and scatter with herbs or garlic for extra flavour.

Substitute sweet potato, yam or taro for white rice or ordinary potato to accompany fish and meat. They can be chopped, boiled and served as they are, or mashed.

Experiment with recipes from other cultures to find new ways of serving root vegetables. Caribbean, African and Middle Eastern cuisines, for example, have interesting and delicious methods of cooking that will revitalise your ideas.

Take advantage of frozen vegetables, which can be cheaper than fresh, and involve no preparation or waste. Unlike canned vegetables, they have no added salt or sugar, and they contain more vitamins and minerals than tired 'fresh' produce.

WHAT IS NSP FIBRE AND WHY IS IT IMPORTANT?

Since the importance of fibre was first recognised in the 1980s when the F-plan diet was popular, it has been realised that fibre encompasses many different types of starch or carbohydrate. It has therefore been renamed non-starchy polysaccharides (NSPs). These different types of starch cannot be digested, so they pass through the gut to the large bowel or colon, where beneficial bacteria ferment them to produce substances that benefit the immune system, help lower cholesterol levels and protect against cancer.

Good sources of NSPs include wholegrain cereals, root vegetables (potato, yam), pulses (beans, lentils, peas) and some fruit (bananas).

3. Vegetable bulbs

Eat as part of the recommended five or more daily portions of fruit and vegetables.

This category includes onions, shallots, chives and garlic, which contain nutrients that have become associated with the prevention of heart disease. In particular, regular consumption of garlic, a characteristic of the Mediterranean diet, is known to help prevent raised blood fats. Similarly, eating raw onion, not something most of us do now, is also associated with heart-health benefits.

Onion, garlic and chives, plus their cousin the leek, contain sulphides that may block the action of cancer-causing chemicals. They also contain quercetin, an antioxidant and anti-inflammatory agent that, like vitamins E and C, appears to be able to mop up potentially harmful free radicals that could otherwise trigger cancer and atherosclerosis (hardening and narrowing of the arteries). Quercetin is also associated with a lower risk of blood-clotting and strokes.

A lower risk of stomach cancer has also been found in a number of countries where people regularly consume relatively large amounts of *alliums* (the Latin name for onion species). The antibacterial effect of garlic may also make stomach ulcers less likely by fighting the bacteria *Helicobacter pylori*, which is associated with them.

Members of the onion family are renowned for adding a pungent flavour to savoury recipes. There is a wide variety of size and colour in onions, from golden-skinned shallots suitable for casseroles and stews, through slender spring onions for salads and stir-fries, to red onions for roasting and making into a savoury 'marmalade'.

Although most often used as one of many ingredients within a recipe, onions are a delicious vegetable in their own right if roasted in their skin and peeled before being served. Spring onions, salad onions and chives are mild enough to eat raw, but they can also be added to stir-fries.

A word of warning about garlic. The bacteria *Clostridium botulinum* is frequently found in soil and sometimes in garlic bulbs. This does not pose a danger unless the garlic is stored in oil in the fridge for more than a day or two, because the low acidity of the oil allows the botulism spores to flourish. For this reason, it is best to use oil flavoured with garlic immediately and not to store it.

Easy ways to eat more bulb vegetables
Make soups based on alliums. The classic French onion soup is satisfying but still reasonably low in fat if you do not add too much cheese (melted on the top). Vichyssoise, based on leeks and potatoes, can be enjoyed hot or cold, and refreshing gazpacho is brimming with raw vegetables, including onion.

Use onions in pizzas and quiches. Pissaladière is a type of pizza tart from southern France based on a delicious thick purée of onions.

Eat more curries and oriental dishes, as many of them contain onions and garlic.

Braise leeks and onions to make a delicious, low-fat vegetable dish. Cook in stock based on mirepoix (a mixture of finely diced carrot, onion and celery) with herbs.

Bake whole leeks under a topping of bread-crumbs and grated cheese to make a gratin.

Accompany offal and lean red meat with onion gravy, made by slowly caramelising sliced onions in minimal fat, then stirring in stock.

Serve red onion marmalade with cold meat, fish, cheese-flavoured and savoury vegetarian dishes. (Soften diced onions in a non-stick pan before adding small amounts of sugar, vinegar, wine and thyme, in which the onion simmers and thickens.)

4. Stalks and stems

Eat as part of the recommended five or more daily portions of fruit and vegetables.

This diverse group has some very tasty members, including asparagus, bamboo shoots, celeriac, celery, fennel, kohlrabi, palm hearts, rhubarb, seakale and Swiss chard (which in some varieties is enjoyed for its large juicy stalks as opposed to its green leaves). All can be cooked and served hot or cold, while some, such as celery and fennel, can be eaten raw. Rhubarb, although technically a vegetable, is sweetened and cooked as a fruit.

The nutritional content of vegetable stalks and stems is impressive, so they are well worth incorporating in your diet. Fennel, for example, contains phyto-oestrogen, while asparagus is an excellent source of folates and vitamin E, and contains NSPs, which promotes the growth of beneficial bacteria in the gut (see probiotics, page 75).

Celery has a long history of being used for medicinal purposes, but is currently in favour for being a very rich source of potassium, vital for regulating blood pressure. The depth of flavour it brings to salads, soups and stews can also help accustom those on low-sodium diets to the reduced salt content of food.

Bamboo shoots may not be eaten frequently, but they are a good source of potassium and very low in calories.

Easy ways to eat more stalks and stems
Roast fennel, lightly brushed with olive oil, or use raw in salads.

Add celery, fennel, kohlrabi and celeriac to slow-cooked casseroles for extra flavour. They go especially well with beans and other pulses that require long, slow cooking.

Make coleslaw more interesting and flavoursome by adding chopped celery. Waldorf salad also benefits from the addition of celery.

Use celeriac to make soups with an excellent celery-like flavour. The benefit over celery is that the slightly starchy texture of celeriac is a natural low-fat thickener, giving a creamy effect without adding cream, butter or eggs.

Serve seakale lightly steamed or 'wilted' with fish.

Incorporate bamboo shoots in stir-fries and Thai vegetable dishes.

Use palm hearts as a crisp addition to salads, or simply steam or stir-fry them.

Cook rhubarb with cinnamon, allspice, ginger or cloves to reduce the sharpness and allow less sugar to be added. You can also combine stewed rhubarb with naturally sweet ingredients, such as ripe strawberries and oranges with ginger, to make delicious compotes.

5. Fruiting vegetables

Eat as part of the recommended five or more daily portions of fruit and vegetables.

Among this group are globe artichokes, aubergines, cauliflowers, courgettes, marrows, peppers, squash and tomatoes. Although we think of them as vegetables and generally use

DAILY VEG

The UK Department of Health recommends eating five portions of fruit and vegetables a day, each portion being roughly equivalent to 80 g/3¼ oz. (You can, of course, eat more if you like. In Australia the government has already 'progressed' to encouraging seven portions a day.)

Vegetable	Portion	Vegetable	Portion
Ackee, canned	3 heaped tbsp	Mange-tout	1 handful
Artichoke	2 globe hearts	Mixed vegetables, frozen	3 tbsp
Asparagus, canned	7 spears	Mushrooms, button	14, or 3 handfuls, or 3–4 heaped tbsp of slices
Asparagus, fresh	5 spears		
Aubergine	¹/₃ of whole		
Beans, black-eyed, cooked	3 heaped tbsp	Mushrooms, dried	2 tbsp or 1 handful porcini
Beans, broad, cooked	3 heaped tbsp		
Beans, butter, cooked	3 heaped tbsp	Okra	16 medium
Beans, cannellini, cooked	3 heaped tbsp	Onions, dried	1 heaped tbsp
Beans, French, cooked	4 heaped tbsp	Onions, fresh	1 medium
Beans, kidney, cooked	3 heaped tbsp	Parsnips	1 large
Beans, runner, cooked	4 heaped tbsp	Peas, canned	3 heaped tbsp
Beansprouts, fresh	2 handfuls	Peas, fresh	3 heaped tbsp
Beetroot, bottled	3 'baby' whole, or 7 slices	Peas, frozen	3 heaped tbsp
		Peas, pigeon, canned	3 heaped tbsp
Broccoli	2 spears	Peas, sugarsnap	1 handful
Brussels sprouts	8	Pepper, canned	½ of whole
Cabbage	¹/₆ small cabbage or 2 handfuls sliced	Pepper, fresh	½ of whole
		Radishes	10
Cabbage, shredded	3 heaped tbsp	Spinach, cooked	2 heaped tbsp
Carrots, canned	3 heaped tbsp	Spinach, fresh	1 cereal bowl
Carrots, fresh, slices	3 heaped tbsp	Spring greens, cooked	4 heaped tbsp
Carrots, shredded	¹/₃ cereal bowl	Spring onions	8 whole
Cauliflower	8 florets	Swede, diced and cooked	3 heaped tbsp
Celery	3 sticks	Sweetcorn, baby	6 whole
Chickpeas	3 heaped tbsp	Sweetcorn, canned	3 heaped tbsp
Chinese leaves	¹/₅ head	Sweetcorn, on the cob	1 cob
Courgettes	½ large courgette	Tomato purée	1 heaped tbsp
Cucumber	5 cm/2 in piece	Tomatoes, fresh	1 medium, or 7 cherry
Curly kale, cooked	4 heaped tbsp		
Karela	½ of whole	Tomatoes, plum, canned	2 whole
Leeks	1 (white parts only)	Tomatoes, sundried	4 pieces
Lentils	3 tbsp		
Lettuce (mixed leaves)	1 cereal bowl		

them for savoury purposes, they are actually fruits.

Globe artichokes are a type of thistle related to the Mediterranean cardoon. The leaves (bracts) that form the choke (flower) each have a fleshy edible base, which softens after boiling. Inside is the 'heart', which can also be eaten. Globe artichokes are a good source of potassium and contain a small amount of calcium, but most of us do not eat them regularly enough for them to have a nutritional impact on our diet.

Aubergines contain useful amounts of potassium and folates, and the deep purple skin contains antioxidant pigments, which are good for the heart.

Red peppers are also rich in antioxidants, and the red and green varieties are high in vitamin C.

Squash, such as the butternut variety, which is a deep orange colour, is a good source of the antioxidant beta-carotene.

Tomatoes are rich in lycopene, an antioxidant found in the red colouring of the skin. This is more available when the fruit is cooked, and seems to have convincing anti-cancer properties and protect against heart disease. Mediterranean men who eat 5–10 servings a week have half the risk of prostate cancer found in other Western men.

Cauliflower is a reasonable source of vitamin C and, as a member of the cabbage family, contains glucosinolates (see page 47).

Courgettes also contribute some vitamin C,

but these and marrows are not hugely nutritious, so just enjoy them for their flavour and low calories.

Easy ways to eat more fruiting vegetables
Use courgettes, marrows and aubergines in curries and casseroles because they absorb the flavours and spices and add texture to sauces.

Make cauliflower cheese using low-fat milk and low-fat cheese.

Sweat tomatoes and courgettes in a covered pan over a low heat, and flavour with basil, marjoram or oregano to make a simple and delicious sauce or side dish.

Serve sauces and salsas based on tomatoes or peppers with meat, fish and vegetarian dishes.

Grill vine tomatoes, or roast them in the oven, brushing with a minimal amount of oil.

Make ratatouille, a versatile Mediterranean vegetable 'stew' containing aubergines, courgettes, peppers and tomatoes. It can be served hot with baked potatoes, or cold as a salad.

Use red peppers to make colourful and flavoursome soups that can be served hot and cold.

Roast whole squash in their skin, then scoop out the flesh and mash.

Stuff peppers, aubergines, courgettes, marrows or large tomatoes with rice or grain mixtures flavoured with herbs and nuts or lean meat.

Add peppers to salads and sandwich fillings.

Top bruschetta (toasted bread brushed with oil and garlic) with sliced or diced tomatoes for a light lunch, snack or starter – or even for breakfast.

6. Pods and seeds

Eat pods as part of the recommended five or more daily portions of fruit and vegetables, and eat seeds several times a week.

A wealth of nutritional benefits can be found in this group, which includes peas, broad beans, runner beans, sprouted beans, such as mung and alfalfa, as well as sweetcorn and the more obvious seeds, such as linseed and sesame seeds.

Peas and beans are familiar to us as fresh vegetables and in their dried form as pulses (see page 69). Both peas and beans are seeds contained in or forming pods. They are usually cooked, although the fresh forms of some peas and beans (not soya beans) may be eaten raw. They contain vitamin C, lots of fibre and more protein than most vegetables. Sprouted seeds contain coumestrol, a potent phyto-oestrogen, but this is most plentiful in sprouted soya beans.

Sweetcorn, although we think of it as a vegetable, is actually the seed of a grass that is classified as a cereal. It is rich in two types of antioxidant carotene – lutein and zeaxanthin – that protect the eyes against age-related

problems, such as cataracts and macular degeneration, the commonest cause of age-related blindness in the West. These types of carotene are also found in red peppers, peas, celery and tomatoes. Sweetcorn is a good source of vitamin C, and it contains a reasonable amount of starchy carbohydrate – for a non-starchy vegetable. It is also a good source of fibre, folates and some B vitamins.

Seeds contain lots of nutrients to fuel the life of a new plant. They are also useful sources of unsaturated fats, and in common with pulses are good vegetable protein foods. If eaten in the correct proportions, they provide vegetarians with the essential amino acids that omnivores or non-vegetarians get from meat, fish, eggs and dairy foods. This is achieved by combining two of the three plant protein food groups: nuts and seeds, pulses (e.g. beans, chickpeas, lentils) and grains (e.g. wheat, oats, barley and rice). However, if you are eating enough calories in a varied diet, you are getting enough protein, and only vegans or others on very restricted diets need to spend time considering combinations of plant protein foods.

Linseed, golden or brown, comes from the flax plant. The whole seeds are rich in omega-3 fats (protective against heart disease) and lignans (beneficial plant hormones with an antioxidant activity, see page 170).

Pumpkin seeds, greenish-grey in colour, are a good source of iron and zinc for a plant food.

Sesame seeds, cream or brown, are rich in unsaturated oils and calcium, and also supply vitamin E and the minerals zinc and iron. They may be eaten roasted or raw, used in sweet or savoury recipes, made into a paste called tahini, or pressed to make sesame oil, which is commonly used in Oriental cooking.

Sunflower seeds, sweet and grey-brown, are a good source of iron, zinc and vitamin C. Once shelled, they can be nibbled as a snack or added to cakes, biscuits, bread and other baked products. They are also a popular ingredient in savoury vegetarian dishes. The oil pressed out of them is rich in polyunsaturates.

Those who avoid dairy products by choice or because of allergy cannot take advantage of the most widely available and richest sources of calcium, but can find adequate amounts in seeds and nuts. For variety, they can also get calcium from wholegrain cereals, oats, pulses, dark green vegetables and dried fruit.

Buy nuts and seeds only from shops that have a regular turnover, and purchase quantities that you will use within a few weeks. All nuts and seeds should be stored in an airtight container in a cool place to prevent the oils in them turning rancid.

Easy ways to eat more seeds
Buy breads and cereals that contain seeds.

Snack on roasted pumpkin seeds and sunflower seeds.

Add pumpkin seeds, sunflower seeds and linseeds to home-made bread dough, and scatter seeds on top of the loaves.

Sprinkle toasted or natural pumpkin seeds and sunflower seeds on salads and fruit salads.

Stir pumpkin seeds, linseeds and sunflower seeds into muesli, or sprinkle over other breakfast cereals.

Add pumpkin seeds and sunflower seeds to vegetarian recipes for roasts, burgers and rissoles.

Include seeds in home-made biscuits, flapjacks and granola bars.

Add poppy seeds to lemon muffins and breads.

Eat hummus, a chickpea dip that contains tahini (sesame seed paste).

Combine sesame seeds with breadcrumbs to make an interesting topping for oven bakes, and a coating for (occasional) fried food.

7. Fruit
Eat as part of the recommended five or more daily portions of fruit and vegetables.

Try to eat all the colours of the rainbow: red from apples, strawberries, raspberries and the blush on many fruits; orange from citrus fruits, mangoes and cantaloupe melon; yellow from starfruit, bananas and grapefruit; green from gooseberries, apples and greengages; indigo from plums and black grapes; violet from blackberries, blueberries and cherries. Of course, there are many other fruits you can eat too.

Fruits provide us with much of our vitamin C and many phytochemicals. Berries, such as blueberries, bilberries, strawberries and raspberries, are rich in ellagic acid, which seems to prevent some carcinogens attacking DNA and causing mutations that can lead to cell division getting out of control. Bilberries also contain bioflavonoids that strengthen cells. The anthocyanins in blueberries, black grapes, cherries and blackcurrants seem to fight cancer and protect against heart disease through their antioxidant and anti-inflammatory properties.

Citrus fruit is best known for its vitamin C content, which fights colds and infections, but it is also a valuable antioxidant that helps protect against cancer and heart disease. Oranges even contain small amounts of iron and folates. The NSP in the pithy part of the fruit is the type that bulks stools and helps speed up transit time.

Prunes are probably better known than oranges for their fibre and usefulness in preventing constipation, but they also are a good source of iron and contribute some selenium.

These are just a few examples of the benefits of having plenty of fruit in your diet. The key is to eat as many types as possible and as frequently as you can.

Can I pop a pill instead of eating all this fruit and veg?

Not really. It might seem like a convenient short cut, but vitamins and minerals work in conjunction with fibre and phyto-chemicals to boost vitality and give protection. It is probably the combination of all these factors that reduces the risk of cancer and heart disease among people who eat a lot of starchy wholegrain foods and fruit and vegetables.

Purified vitamins and minerals in pill form cannot offer the same sort of advantage. And, in fact, the government has advised people against taking certain supplements, such as beta-carotene, because some studies have

DAILY FRUIT

The UK Department of Health recommends eating five portions of fruit and vegetables a day, each portion being roughly equivalent to 80 g/3¼ oz. (You can, of course, eat more if you like. In Australia the government has already 'progressed' to encouraging seven portions a day.)

Fruit	Portion
Apples, dried rings	4
Apples, fresh	1 medium
Apples, puréed	2 heaped tbsp
Apricots, canned	6 halves
Apricots, dried	3 whole
Apricots, fresh	3 apricots
Apricots, ready to eat	3 whole
Avocado	½ of whole
Banana, chips	1 handful
Bananas, fresh	1 medium
Blackberries	1 handful (9–10 berries)
Blackcurrants	4 heaped tbsp
Blueberries	2 handfuls (4 heaped tbsp)
Cherries, canned	11 cherries (3 heaped tbsp)
Cherries, dried	1 heaped tbsp
Cherries, fresh	14
Clementines	2
Currants, dried	1 heaped tbsp
Damsons	5–6
Dates, fresh	3
Fig, dried	2
Fig, fresh	2
Fruit juice	150 ml/5 fl oz
Fruit salad, canned	3 heaped tbsp
Fruit salad, fresh	3 heaped tbsp
Fruit smoothie	150 ml/5 fl oz
Gooseberries	1 handful
Grapefruit, canned	3 heaped tbsp (8 segments)
Grapefruit segments, fresh	½ of whole fruit
Grapes	1 handful
Kiwi fruit	2
Kumquats	6–8
Lychees, canned	6
Lychees, fresh	6

Fruit	Portion
Mandarin oranges, canned	3 heaped tbsp
Mandarin oranges, fresh	1 medium
Mango	2 slices (5 cm/2 in thick)
Melon	1 slice (5 cm/2 in thick)
Mixed fruit, dried	1 heaped tbsp
Nectarines	1
Orange	1
Passion fruit	5–6 fruits
Pawpaw (papaya), fresh	1 slice
Peach, canned	2 halves or 7 slices
Peach, dried	2 halves
Peach, fresh	1 medium
Peach, ready to eat	2 halves
Pears, canned	2 halves or 7 slices
Pears, dried	2 halves
Pears, fresh	1 medium pear
Pears, ready to eat	2 halves
Pineapple, canned	2 rings or 12 chunks
Pineapple, crushed	3 tbsp
Pineapple, dried	1 heaped tbsp
Pineapple, fresh	1 large slice
Plums, fresh	2 medium
Prunes, canned	6
Prunes, dried	3
Prunes, ready to eat	3
Raisins	1 tbsp
Raspberries, canned	20 raspberries
Raspberries, fresh	2 handfuls
Rhubarb, canned	5 chunks
Rhubarb, cooked	2 heaped tbsp
Satsumas	2 small
Sharon fruit	1
Strawberries, canned	9
Strawberries, fresh	7
Sultanas	1 heaped tbsp
Tangerines	2 small

suggested they can increase the risk of lung cancer in smokers. Taking moderate to high doses of any vitamin or mineral cannot be assumed to be risk free.

Nonetheless, as very few people reach the target of eating enough fruit and vegetables, and as other areas of their diet are also imperfect, there is an argument to say that multivitamin and mineral supplements could have a role to play in fighting chronic diseases such as heart disease and cancer. Indeed, researchers at Harvard Medical School in 2002 concluded that as 'Inadequate intake of several vitamins has been linked to chronic diseases, including coronary heart disease, cancer and osteoporosis...we recommend that all adults take one multivitamin daily.'

If you take their advice, choose a product that offers around 100 per cent of the recommended daily amount (RDA); don't go mad with mega-doses.

HOW TO FIT IN FIVE A DAY

Here are some examples of how you could fit five portions of fruit and vegetables into a normal day's healthy eating.

Breakfast – bowl of cereal with skimmed or semi-skimmed milk and 1 tablespoonful of dried fruit, such as raisins, apricots or prunes (1 portion)

Lunch – tuna salad sandwich ($\frac{1}{2}$ portion, as you can't fit much salad, grated carrot or sliced pepper in a sandwich); yoghurt and fresh fruit, such as an apple, pear or banana (1 portion)

TOP-SCORING ANTIOXIDANT FRUIT AND VEGETABLES

It's not really known how the test-tube anti-oxidant performance of various fruits and vegetables translates into 'real life', that is, the effect they have in your body when eaten. However, the fruits and vegetables themselves make delicious additions to your diet, and it is known that diets rich in these foods generally lower the risk of chronic disease.

The oxygen radical absorbance capacity (ORAC) score relates to the total antioxidant power of food. The amounts are units per 100 g/4 oz of food.

Fruit	ORAC	Vegetable	ORAC
Prunes	5770	Kale	1770
Raisins	2830	Spinach	1260
Blueberries	2400	Brussels sprouts	980
Blackberries	2036	Alfalfa sprouts	930
Strawberries	1540	Broccoli	890
Raspberries	1220	Beets	840
Plums	949	Red peppers	710
Oranges	750	Onions	450
Red grapes	739	Sweetcorn	400
Cherries	670	Aubergines	390
Kiwi fruit	602		
Pink grapefruit	483		

Source: Based on research by the Human Nutrition Research Center on Aging, Tufts University, Boston, USA (1997)

Main meal – grilled chicken breast with rice or baked potato and 3 tablespoonfuls of mixed vegetables (1 portion); glass of tomato juice (1 portion); large slice of melon for pudding (1 portion)

Total: 5$\frac{1}{2}$ portions

Here's another typical day
Breakfast: - boiled or poached egg with wholegrain bread and spread
Snack – piece of fruit (1 portion)

Lunch – bowl of pasta in tomato or non-creamy vegetable sauce (1 portion) with side salad (1 portion) and dressing, if liked

Main meal – reduced-fat sausages with mashed potato or oven chips, with 1 corn on the cob or 3 heaped tablespoons sweetcorn or 6 baby corn (1 portion) and 1 grilled tomato or 6 cherry tomatoes (1 portion); apple or rhubarb crumble (1 portion) with low-fat yoghurt or custard.
Total: 6 portions

8. Whole wheat
Eat as part of the recommended 6–11 daily portions of starchy carbohydrate foods.

As a wholegrain food, whole wheat contains all parts of the grain – the outer bran layer, the starchy centre and the germ or seed. While the individual parts are all beneficial, it is the combination of all three working together that makes whole grains so valuable. Refined products, even if fibre (usually in the form of bran) has been added, are less beneficial.

Until recently the fibre content of whole grains, which has anti-cancer properties and protects against heart disease, was thought to be the main source of benefit, but now it seems that the minerals, vitamins, antioxidants and other phytochemicals also play an important part. Plant sterols found in whole grains and seeds have been shown to lower cholesterol if eaten in large enough quantities (and are added to cholesterol-lowering food products, such as spreads and desserts). Whole grains are also rich in oligosaccharides, a type of NSP fermented by beneficial bacteria in the gut, which seems to help lower serum cholesterol and may have an anti-cancer role. Wholegrain wheat also contains plant oestrogens and lignans, which have anti-cancer properties.

The main problem with refined carbohydrates, such as white bread, sugary breakfast cereals, cakes, biscuits and syrups, is that they are very easily digested, having the effect of raising levels of LDL (bad) cholesterol and lowering levels of HDL (good) cholesterol, which increases the risk of heart disease. The rapid digestion of refined carbohydrates also causes blood sugar to rise very fast and large quantities of insulin to be released. This is particularly problematic if you are overweight, inactive and susceptible to type 2 diabetes (see Metabolic Syndrome, page 36). Replacing as much highly refined (often high-fat) carbohydrate food as possible with wholegrain and unrefined starchy carbohydrates avoids risking your health on the damaging sugar-insulin roller-coaster.

Wheat is the principal grain in the UK, and most wholegrain foods, including bread, pasta, breakfast cereals and baked goods, are made from it. Wholegrain wheat products and refined white flour products contain similar amounts of protein, but the benefits of whole wheat lie more in its content of fibre, iron and vitamins B_1, B_2 and B_3. Although most of the wheat we eat is processed to some degree, wheat berries (grains) can be bought from health food shops and prepared and eaten like rice.

Bread is a staple part of the Western diet, and eating it regularly, especially in wholegrain varieties, is a good idea. The best choices are multigrain breads, which contain whole and kibbled (coarsely ground) grains, including wheat, barley, oats and oat bran, and pumpernickel, a wholemeal rye bread. Light rye breads, sourdough, brown, white and wholemeal loaves contain less whole grain, but are still good choices for variety. Very dark rye bread and black bread (not pumpernickel) have a high glycaemic index (see page 168), so are not the best choices. Baguettes and bagels are very refined white breads, and offer little in the way of nutrients.

Pasta, particularly the wholemeal variety, is a healthy fast food, whether dried or fresh. Although primarily a starchy food, it is also a good source of fibre, protein and vitamins B_1, B_2 and B_3. When made from traditional durum wheat, which contains a hard type of starch that releases its energy in a steady stream, causing little disruption to blood-sugar levels, pasta has a beneficial low glycaemic index (see page 169).

The germ (seed) found at the base of the wheat grain is packed with nutrients to feed an embryonic plant. This rich source of polyunsaturated fat, protein and vitamins B_1, B_2, B_3 and E is milled into soft, creamy flakes and sold as wheatgerm. Eaten straight from the pack, it contains 2–2.5 g of fibre per 100 g, the same amount found in white bread, and its vitamin E content (hard to come by in other foods) makes it a valuable addition to the diet.

Sometimes wheatgerm is 'stabilised', which

WHOLEGRAIN LABELLING

Manufacturers define wholegrain foods as those in which 51 per cent or more of the ingredients are whole grains. This means that whole grains will be the first item on the food label because ingredients are listed in descending order of quantity. Check this out next time you buy crispbread, breakfast cereal, bread, rice or pasta.

means that it has been mildly heat-treated. This loses a few of the vitamins, but not enough to worry about. However, do not be tempted to buy defatted wheatgerm, even though it has a long shelf life: removing the fat also removes most of the nutrients. Wheatgerm should be stored in an airtight container and refrigerated after opening to prevent its natural oils becoming rancid.

'Bran' usually means wheat bran in the UK, although oat and rice brans are also sold in healthfood shops. However, it is better to eat the whole grain than add bran to refined white foods because the whole grain contains more fibre and minerals. In addition, the processing and cooking of wholegrain products seems to increase the availability of the minerals. Bran also contains phytate, a substance that binds minerals, such as iron, making them unavailable to the body. However, a beneficial role for phytates in fighting disease is emerging.

Some refined forms of wheat, although less nutritious than the whole grain, can make useful additions to the diet.

Bulgur is kibbled (cracked) wheat grain that has been partially cooked. It can also be found under other names, such as burghul, bulghul, pilgouri and pourgouri. In the Middle East it is widely eaten in place of rice, added to soups, or forms the basis of a refreshing salad called tabbouleh, in which it is mixed with chopped cucumber, mint and lemons.

The protein content of bulgur is similar to that of oats, but higher than in barley and buckwheat, and the fat content is lower than most other grains. It is a good source of calcium, matching whole wheat, but with slightly less iron. Like other whole grains, bulgur also provides reasonable amounts of vitamins B_1, B_2 and B_3.

Couscous is a partially cooked grain made from rolled semolina, the inside of the wheat grain. (Barley and millet varieties are also available.) The process of refining makes it far lower in fibre than the whole grain, but it still contains 5 per cent, and has a protein content to match the wheat from which it is produced. In general, the vitamin and mineral content is more than halved by the processing.

Even though couscous and bulgur are lower in nutrients than whole wheat, they make interesting additions to the diet, and since recipes using them frequently contain vegetables, they may also help to increase vegetable intake.

Easy ways to eat more whole wheat
Cut thick slices from your loaf, or choose thick-cut sliced bread.

Top up your wholegrain intake with bread if

HOW MANY PORTIONS OF STARCHY FOODS DO YOU NEED?

The daily recommended intake of starchy foods is 6–11 portions. This might seem rather a wide variation, but it is designed to accommodate the different needs of different age groups and lifestyles.

Age	Active women	Sedentary women
11–14	7–9	5–7
15–18	9–11	6–8
19–49	8–10	6–8
50+	6–8	6–8

Age	Active men	Sedentary men
11–14	9–11	7–9
15–18	10–14	9–10
19–49	10–11	8–10
50–65	7–10	7–10
65+	6–8	6–8

you do not eat other wholegrain foods. (To keep calories down, don't use butter or spread, especially in sandwiches with moist fillings.)

Make a meal of toasted sandwiches with salad and coleslaw.

Replace biscuits, cakes and other refined snacks with low-sugar and low-fat wholemeal buns.

Eat wholewheat pasta rather than the white varieties. (Those intolerant of the gluten in wheat can eat pasta or noodles made from rice flour, vegetable flour, or soya and mung bean flours. The bean products have a particularly low glycaemic index, see page 169.)

Use leftover pasta to make salads for packed lunches.

Make stir-fries using high-fibre noodles.

Serve wholewheat pasta as a starter to special occasion meals (when you are not slimming).

Add wheatgerm to crumble toppings, scones, bread, biscuits and cakes when you are baking.

Eat more Hovis and other 'wheatgerm' breads.

Sprinkle wheatgerm over breakfast cereal or stir into muesli.

Use wheatgerm as a binder or filler in home-made meatloaf and burgers, or vegetarian equivalents made from lentil and wholegrain mixtures; it is not intrusive in texture or flavour.

Coat food such as fishcakes and rissoles with a mixture of wheatgerm, herbs and spices instead of breadcrumbs.

Sprinkle wheatgerm over yoghurt or other desserts as a topping.

9. Other whole grains
Eat as part of the recommended 6–11 daily portions of starchy carbohydrate foods.

The health benefits of wheat, the most common whole grain, have been discussed in section 8. Here we look at some of the more unusual whole grains, which bring many of the same benefits, and also add variety and interest to your diet.

Barley is a nutritious grain with high levels of protein and iron, but most of the UK production goes into animal foods and the brewing industry. Probably the best-known barley product is malt extract, a dietary supplement and food ingredient. 'Pearl' barley, the form in which it is traditionally added as a bulking agent to soups and stews, is only the inner part of the grain. Thus the high-fibre value of the whole grain is lost, and the iron, calcium and B vitamin content (similar to that of oats) is halved by the processing. Slightly more nutrients are retained in the less refined 'pot' barley and barley flakes, which are sold alongside whole barley grains in some healthfood shops. The grains can be boiled, like rice, although they take longer to cook (around 40 minutes). They contain lignans and other beneficial phytochemicals.

The soluble types of fibre in barley are similar to those in oats, but as we eat so little barley, we do not benefit from them.

Buckwheat is the tiny dark seed of a non-cereal Chinese plant, so strictly speaking it is not a grain. However, it is ground into flour and used to make pancakes, such as Breton crêpes, and certain Japanese noodles. It is also used in gluten-free flour mixes.

Buckwheat has a high protein content, and is especially rich in one of the amino acids (protein building blocks) that is low in other grains.

Buckwheat groats, the crushed form of the

grain, are sold roasted and unroasted in healthfood shops. When boiled in twice their volume of water, the cooked grains (called *kasha* in Russia) can be mixed with nuts, vegetables or meat to make pilaf, used as a stuffing for cabbage, or combined in meatballs. Kasha can also be sweetened for breakfast, or served plain instead of potatoes or rice.

Corn is more familiar in the UK as sweetcorn or corn on the cob than in its dried version, which is classified as a cereal. The correct name for corn is maize, and the dried kernels are milled to make cornmeal (the main ingredient in polenta), cornflour and grits, which are all suitable for gluten-free diets.

Cornmeal is only a moderate source of protein. It contains fewer B vitamins than other cereals, and its vitamin B_3 is biologically unavailable until the grain has been heat-treated with lime in an alkaline solution. This is vital in countries where corn is a staple food. The Aztecs and Native Americans, who relied on corn, used to eat it in combination with beans and squash to make up for its nutritional deficiencies. Nowadays, calcium is added during the processing for the same purpose.

The germ of corn contains a large amount of polyunsaturated fat, which is processed into corn oil for cooking and salad dressings.

Millet is a gluten-free, nutty yellow grain, which can be served in place of rice or potatoes. In Africa, where it is a staple food, the whole grains are roughly crushed to a flour and mixed with water to make porridge, or slightly fermented and made into flat breads.

In the UK millet is sold in healthfood shops. It cooks quickly and can be used to make tabbouleh-style salads. It is high in fibre, contains a good amount of protein, and has an unsaturated fat content on a par with oats. Millet also contains useful amounts of zinc, iron and vitamin B_3 and E.

Oats are a whole grain because the milling process is not very intensive and preserves a high percentage of their nutrients. After the outer husk is removed, the inner groat is ground and cut into pieces known as pinhead meal, which is ground further to make oatmeal, from which porridge and biscuits can be made. For porridge oats the groats are steamed and rolled flat between heavy rollers, which inactivates the enzymes that cause the natural oils to go rancid, thus lengthening the shelf life. When large groats are rolled, the result is jumbo oats. Oat flakes made from pinhead meal are quicker to cook.

Studies have shown that regularly eating oats as part of a low-fat balanced diet can help reduce cholesterol levels. The effective amount is 125–150 g/4–5 oz per day, which is quite a lot of oats, as you get about 40–50 g/ 1½–2 oz in a medium bowl of porridge, a large flapjack or an oatmeal muffin. (Flapjacks are, of course, high in calories, fat and sugar, as are most muffins, so these are suitable only for very active people without a weight problem.) In fact, oats exert a small beneficial effect (most clearly seen in people with raised cholesterol levels) even when the intake is as little as 40–50 g/1½–2 oz a day.

The constituent responsible for reducing both total blood cholesterol and levels of harmful

LDL without reducing levels of protective HDL is one of the soluble types of fibre. This is also associated with lower blood pressure and a reduced risk of colon cancer, especially when oats form part of a high-fibre diet.

For a cereal, oats contain a high level of fat (5–9 per cent), but this is beneficial because the fat is unsaturated. Oats are also a good source of protein, iron, calcium and some B vitamins, including certain folates.

Blood-sugar levels rise very slowly after eating oats, so they provide a steady stream of energy and are especially useful for diabetics. Since oats are filling and low-calorie, they can also help people trying to lose weight.

Oats are gluten-free, so in theory they are suitable for people with coeliac disease. However, they contain a protein similar to gluten, which means that some patients cannot tolerate them.

Quinoa, a Peruvian grain that looks like pinkish-brown millet and is related to spinach, has been grown in the Andes since Inca times. It has a delicate flavour and smooth texture. Quinoa is very high in protein, and matches oats for its unsaturated fat content, which is a good source of vitamin E. The iron content is the highest among whole grains, and it also contains good amounts of zinc and calcium, folates and vitamins B_1 and B_2.

Quinoa, which is gluten-free, can be used in place of rice or potatoes, or used in salads and stuffings. Look out for quinoa in specialist breakfast cereals. Its flour may also be used in baked goods.

Rye is milled to make bread flour, but is usually mixed with wheat flour because it is low in gluten, which is necessary for making dough rise. On its own, it is used to make pumpernickel, a dense, dark bread. As a general rule, the darker the bread, the higher the fibre content. Rye is often the basis of sourdough breads, which use a fermented starter rather than baker's yeast as a raising agent, and have a characteristic flavour. We are also familiar with rye in crispbreads and crackers.

Studies of people who habitually eat dark rye breads (which also often contain barley and sometimes oats) show lower rates of heart disease, possibly because of the cholesterol-lowering effect of the fibre in which they are rich. Rye also contains very high levels of the mineral selenium, an important antioxidant associated with lower risks of cancer, and high levels of vitamin E. Other potential anti-cancer benefits in rye include protease inhibitors, which block the action of enzymes known to promote growth in cancer cells.

Rye is also a reasonable source of iron and some B vitamins. In its wholegrain form, it is used mainly for fermenting into malted whisky and other drinks. However, rye flakes are often added to multigrain breads, and rye flour can be used for bread-making at home.

Triticale is a hybrid of wheat and rye. Resembling dark-coloured long-grain rice, it has a chewy texture and earthy taste. It is sold in healthfood shops and can be boiled like any other whole grain, and used in place of rice and potatoes. Look out for it in flaked form in specialist breakfast cereals.

Triticale has a moderate vitamin E content, and amounts of unsaturated fat similar to those in other whole grains. It is a good source of zinc and contains reasonable quantities of iron and calcium. The fibre content is high, probably somewhere between rye and wheat.

Easy ways to eat more whole grains
Cut back on refined (white) versions of staple foods and make more use of bulgur, couscous, millet, quinoa and wheat berries.

Use pumpernickel bread to make open sandwiches topped with prawns, or lean ham, and plenty of salad and raw vegetables.

Cut thicker slices of wholegrain bread, or buy thick-cut varieties.

Choose breads that contain whole grains, kibbled grains or flaked grains, such as barley, oats and rye.

Snack on wholegrain, low-fat treats instead of refined cakes, biscuits and confectionery.

Consult a good Middle Eastern cookery book to find lots of delicious ways to use bulgur and couscous.

Fill tortillas and taco shells with salad and beans for a satisfying lunch or supper.

Serve tortillas or tacos with meat mixtures, such as chilli con carne.

Eat corn chips with vegetable dips, such as tomato salsa and guacamole.

Have 'wrap'-style sandwiches for packed lunches.

Serve polenta with lean red meat dishes.

Grill sliced polenta topped with cheese and serve with salads.

Make regular use of oat-based breakfast cereals, such as porridge, muesli and granola.

Add oats to home-made bread – about 40 g/1½ oz oats to 400 g/14 oz of flour.

Eat oatcakes rather than crackers as a savoury snack on their own or with cheese.

Buy oatmeal varieties of sweet biscuits.

Choose cakes and snack bars (if you must) that contain a generous amount of oats.

10. Breakfast cereal
Eat as part of the recommended 6–11 daily portions of starchy carbohydrate foods.

The ideal breakfast should be mainly carbohydrate, namely, starchy foods, such as bread and cereal, to raise blood-sugar levels after the night's fast. Wholegrain cereal, such as shredded wheat or wholewheat breakfast 'biscuits', is a better choice for everyday eating than a refined (white) cereal that may be frosted or have sugary additions, such as chocolate or toffee, because it releases energy slowly, contains more fibre and nutrients, and usually less sugar. Along with porridge, prunes and other dried fruit, wholegrain cereals increase the fibre content of breakfast, which helps to lower cholesterol levels. However, sugary cereals can be eaten occasionally for variety, and it's better to eat them (especially fortified ones) than to skip breakfast entirely.

Choosing a fortified breakfast cereal helps you receive the recommended daily amount of nutrients that may be in short supply, such as iron and folic acid. Folic acid reduces the risk of heart disease and protects unborn babies against spina bifida.

Cornflakes are one of the most popular breakfast cereals, but they are high in sodium, which is bad for blood pressure (see page 24). If you particularly like the taste of corn, choose lower-sodium types of corn-based cereals instead.

The milk poured over the cereal is a good source of vitamin B_{12}, which is needed to work with folic acid to lower homocysteine levels to protect against heart disease. The milk also provides protein and calcium for strong bones. (If you prefer soya milk, choose a fortified low-sugar version.)

In general, breakfast is a good habit to have because if it is skipped, the missed nutrients are rarely made up during the day. In addition, breakfast-eaters perform better in their daily tasks and are generally more successful at weight control.

Easy ways to eat more breakfast cereal
Take it to work if you do not have time for breakfast.

Use cereals as a snack at any time of day.

Top yoghurt and fruit compotes with crunchy cereals, such as granola or flakes.

Serve cereal as an after-school or after-work snack.

11. Rice

Eat as part of the recommended 6–11 daily portions of starchy carbohydrate foods.

Available in many varieties, rice is the staple food of more than half the world's population. The best choice for increasing wholegrain intake is brown rice.

All varieties of rice have the inedible husk removed after harvesting. Brown rice retains the bran layer and germ, but to produce white rice these are removed. Consequently, brown rice is richer in nutrients, especially vitamins B_1, B_2, B_3, B_6 and E, fibre and potassium.

'Easycook' brown rice has been steeped in hot water and partially steamed, which retains nutrients from the bran layer in the grain, but it is not as nutritious as the unrefined variety.

White rice varieties, whether long-grain, such as basmati, or short-grain, such as arborio and carnaroli (used for risotto), glutinous (sticky) and 'instant' (quick-cook), have been further refined and are not whole grains. These are basically just sources of energy, but nice for a change. White rice is particularly low in vitamin B_1 and other B vitamins, leading to deficiency diseases among people who over-rely on it.

Wild rice, the seed of an aquatic grass, is brown-black in colour, more elongated and chewier than long-grain white rice, and has a distinctive nutty flavour. Like rice, it is gluten-free, but it contains almost twice as much protein, iron, calcium and folates as brown rice, making it very nutritious. Its vitamin B_1 content is lower than brown rice, however, but higher than white.

Easy ways to eat more rice

Serve rice instead of potatoes or pasta. (Rice is particularly useful for those intolerant of wheat or who have coeliac disease because it is gluten-free.)

Make more rice dishes, such as kedgerees, pilaus, paellas, risottos, biryanis and pilafs.

Increase the portion size when serving rice.

Serve wholegrain rice breakfast cereals.

Try ground brown rice as a breakfast 'porridge'.

Make rice rather than meat or fish the main part of a meal.

Add rice to soups.

Use cold cooked rice to make salads.

Snack on plain, sweet or savoury rice cakes.

12. Nuts

Eat at least several times a week.

Almonds, brazils, cashews, hazelnuts, macadamia nuts, peanuts, pecans, pistachios and walnuts – virtually all nuts are good sources of fibre and are rich in unsaturated fats. The exceptions are coconut, which is high in saturated fat, and chestnuts, which (unlike other nuts) lack beneficial omega-3 acids and are low in protein, but are rich in carbohydrate.

As there is such a wide choice of nuts, and they are so versatile in sweet and savoury dishes, and as snacks, it is relatively easy to make them a regular part of your diet. Eating nuts four or five times a week is associated with a much lower risk of heart disease. In fact it may be nuts rather than wine (see page 28) that should be credited for the French paradox in the Mediterranean diet, namely the fact that the French eat lots of fatty food but have far less heart disease than the British. Perhaps the plant sterols in nuts that the French consume regularly, like the phenols in wine, help lower cholesterol levels.

Clinical studies have shown that diets supplemented with walnuts, almonds, peanuts or macadamia nuts decrease levels of cholesterol, particularly harmful LDL cholesterol, lowering the risk of heart attacks. This is due to the nuts' unsaturated fat content. Most nuts are also rich in arginine, an amino acid from which nitric oxide is made, and this is known to protect against heart disease. The other potentially protective constituents of nuts include magnesium, which helps to regulate heart beat and muscle contraction, folates, which reduce homocysteine levels (see page 24), copper, an antioxidant mineral, potassium, which regulates blood pressure, fibre and vitamin E, food sources of which are associated with lower heart disease.

Specific 'good guys' include walnuts, which are especially high in unsaturated omega-3 fats, brazil nuts, which are a rich source of the antioxidant mineral selenium (a protector against cancer and often lacking in the UK diet), and peanuts (actually pulses rather than nuts because they grow underground). Peanuts are highly nutritious in any form, but

NUTS: THE INSIDE STORY

100 g/4 oz	Calories	Total fat	Saturates	Monoun-saturates	Polyun-saturates	Protein	Fibre
Almonds	565	53.6	8.3	71.6	19.6	16.9	14.3
Brazils	619	61.5	26.7	34.3	39.0	12.0	9.0
Cashews	561	45.7	17.5	70.0	6.5	17.2	1.4
Chestnuts	170	2.7	18.2	39.2	41.9	2.0	6.8
Coconut, fresh	351	36.0	83.0	7.0	1.8	3.2	13.6
Hazelnuts	380	36.0	7.2	81.7	10.9	7.6	6.1
Peanuts	570	49.0	15.2	50.1	29.8	24.3	8.1
Pecans	687	71.2	7.0	63.2	19.6	9.2	2.3
Pistachios	594	53.7	9.3	65.1	18.6	19.3	1.9
Walnuts	525	51.5	11.4	16.3	71.4	10.6	5.2

when buying peanut butter choose varieties that are low in salt and saturated fats.

The benefits of eating nuts do not, however, give you carte blanche to eat bag after bag of them in the pub or wine bar. Apart from the salt content being harmful, nuts are high in calories because they are rich in fat, albeit beneficial fats. Therefore, they are best eaten as the protein part of a main meal rather than a between-meal snack for people who are overweight or dieting. Nuts and nut-based recipes make a good substitute for protein foods that are high in saturated fats, such as sausages and meat pies.

Easy ways to eat more nuts
Add nuts to home-made bread. Walnuts, pecans and hazelnuts are particularly successful.

Make cakes that are based on ground almonds rather than flour.

Chop nuts and sprinkle them on wholegrain breakfast cereals, yoghurt and other low-fat dairy desserts. Toasted hazelnuts and almonds are particularly tasty.

Add nuts to main meal salads to provide a healthier source of protein than pork pies or Scotch eggs, for example. The nuts also contain fibre, which is lacking in animal protein.

Serve pasta with pesto, a simple sauce made from ground pine nuts, olive oil, basil leaves and Parmesan cheese.

Experiment with recipes for nut roasts and burgers – they're better than they sound – and serve with salad.

13. Pulses
Eat at least several times a week.

Also known as legumes, this group of key foods includes dried beans, peas and lentils. They are an excellent source of virtually fat-free protein, fibre, vitamins B_1, B_2 and B_3, calcium, zinc and iron. In addition, they include a good range of minerals – magnesium, phosphorus, potassium, copper, manganese and selenium – and contain lots of phytonutrients that help lower cholesterol levels, control blood-sugar levels and protect against cancer and osteoporosis. They also contain inhibitors of enzymes linked to tumour growth, and help prevent cell reproduction in the intestine, which may protect against colon cancer.

Isoflavones, a type of plant oestrogen found in pulses, have been associated with a lower risk of cancer, particularly breast and prostate cancers. As oestrogen promotes bone health, foods rich in isoflavones are also seen to help protect against osteoporosis.

It is better to eat isoflavones in food than in supplements because the foods that contain them are also rich in fibre, protein and other nutrients. Healthy intakes for different age groups are being researched, but in the West we eat less than 1 mg a day, compared with up to 50 mg in China and Japan. Pulses also contain other types of phyto-oestrogen: coumestrol and lignans.

The greatest health benefits from phyto-oestrogens seem to be gained by those who eat them regularly throughout life, but they are worth including in your diet even if you're only just starting to eat them.

Buy pulses from a shop with a good turnover because the older they are, the tougher and drier they become, the longer they take to cook and the lower their nutritional content.

The soluble types of fibre in pulses are also associated with a lower risk of heart disease because, when eaten daily, or several times a week, they help lower cholesterol. Soya protein has a similar effect. Pulses also have a low glycaemic index (see page 169), so blood-sugar levels rise slowly and steadily after they have been eaten. This is beneficial for most people, but diabetics in particular.

Traditional use of pulses with cereals in combinations such as beans on toast, dhal or curry with rice or bread, and Caribbean rice with peas makes nutritional sense because the two different types of foods make up for each other's amino acid (protein) deficiencies to improve the quality of the protein.

Know your pulses

There are many different types of pulse, which share the general nutritional benefits outlined earlier, so make regular use of as many as possible to create a healthy diet. If buying canned pulses, be aware that they are high in sodium, so choose varieties without added salt.

Aduki (or adzuki) beans are small and either dark red or yellow. They can be cooked and used in soups, stews, curries and salads. They are also ideal for sprouting. Sprouted seeds have the advantage of containing vitamin C, not found in dried pulses. Aduki beans contain more zinc than most other pulses.

Chickpeas, the basis of hummus, felafel, and other Middle Eastern dishes, are rich in lignans, a type of phyto-oestrogen. They also contain antioxidant saponins. The saponins' ability to bind cholesterol in the gut reduces the amount of cholesterol absorbed into the bloodstream. Another role of saponins is to stimulate the immune system and inhibit cancer cell development.

The soluble fibre in chickpeas helps lower cholesterol by removing it from the body, while another type of NSP (oligosaccharides) supports beneficial gut bacteria.

Chickpeas are a good source of selenium as well as the other minerals associated with pulses.

Gram flour made from chickpeas contains a greater concentration of nutrients than cooked chickpeas. It is used to make nutritious Indian pancakes, which can be filled with vegetable mixtures and served with raw and cooked vegetable relishes (sambals). The flour is rich in protein, calcium, magnesium, iron, zinc, potassium and some B vitamins.

Haricot beans are used to make the baked beans that we're so familiar with, and the classic French cassoulet. They are particularly rich in calcium, potassium, iron and zinc.

Lentils are a good source of fibre, lignans and selenium. All varieties contain reasonable amounts of iron, potassium, magnesium and some B vitamins (but not B$_{12}$). However, green and brown lentils have slightly higher levels than the split orange and red varieties.

Mung beans are small, dark green beans, more familiar in their sprouted form as white beansprouts, which contain vitamin C and are rich in the phyto-oestrogen coumestrol.

Soya beans are not a traditional part of the Western diet, but products such as soya milk and soya-based meat substitutes are well known and increasingly available. Soya protein, in amounts of 25–50 g/1–2 oz a day, has been shown to lower total and LDL cholesterol when used in conjunction with a low-fat diet. In the UK and USA cholesterol-lowering claims are allowed on foods that supply 25 g/1 oz of soya protein a day.

It has been estimated that regular consumption of soya could reduce the risk of heart disease by up to 40 per cent. If buying soya foods or soya milk, look for varieties that are low in sugar and fat. Some soya milks are fortified with calcium so that they make a nutritional contribution similar to cows' milk.

Soya beans are the richest source of isoflavones, the benefits of which have been discussed earlier. Isoflavones are not destroyed by the heat and processing involved in making soya products, but the amounts of protein and isoflavones will vary between brands. Some estimates say that around 40 mg of isoflavones per day (the equivalent of 100 g/4 oz of cooked soya beans) could supply the benefits of a traditional healthy Japanese diet.

Tofu (soya bean curd) is made by soaking, grinding and boiling soya beans. The resulting soya milk is then turned into a curd by adding a mineral coagulant (calcium and/or magnesium sulphate), and the curd is pressed into blocks. The calcium and magnesium content depends on the method of production, and can range from 32 mg of calcium per 100 g/4 oz to 683 mg in the same quantity; magnesium variation is far less.

Tofu is a low-fat protein food, but the protein content varies between types of tofu (silken, firm, extra firm) and brands, so read the label. The fat in tofu is mainly unsaturated (as it is in soya beans, which go to make soya oil). Tofu contains some iron, zinc and small amounts of B vitamins, except vitamin B_{12}.

Available plain, flavoured or smoked, tofu contains around 8 per cent protein and 3.5 per cent fat. Firm tofu can be marinated to improve the flavour, barbecued, grilled or steamed. Soft tofu can be scrambled and used in dressings, sauces and dairy-free cheesecakes.

Tempeh is another soya-based protein alternative, containing about 20 per cent protein, 3 per cent fat and good amounts of vitamin B. It contains less calcium and magnesium than some tofu, but useful amounts nonetheless. It is made by boiling the beans, then incubating them with a special bacteria. The resulting 'cake' of tempeh smells a bit like mushrooms and can be sliced, diced or shaped for use in lots of vegetarian and vegan recipes.

Easy ways to eat more pulses
Make beans on toast, or use beans as a baked potato filling; choose lower salt versions.

Eat pulse-based curries, such as dhal (lentils).

Extend meat dishes by adding pulses, e.g. chilli con carne.
Make pulses the basis of soups and stews.

Try vegetarian pâtés and burgers, low-fat versions of the meat-based types.

Go Mexican with tacos and refried beans.

Use tofu and tempeh in stir-fries and other oriental recipes.

Add beans and chickpeas to salads as the main protein ingredient.

14. Fats and oils
Limit your intake and choose the right kind.

Over-consumption of fat, particularly saturated fat (lard, butter, ghee, block margarine and cooking fats), is one of the major causes of chronic health problems.

The maximum amount of fat needed depends on age, body size and activity levels. To maintain a healthy weight if leading a sedentary lifestyle, women should eat no more than 70 g/2¾ oz of fat a day, and men no more than 90 g/3½ oz.

Cutting down on saturates means swapping from lard, butter, ghee and solid margarine to unsaturated fats that contain monounsaturated or polyunsaturated fatty acids. Polyunsaturated oils include sunflower, groundnut, soya and safflower, which are neutral in flavour and colour. They supply the essential fatty acids (EFAs) omega-3 and omega-6, fat-soluble vitamin E, an antioxidant necessary for cell structure. Fat spreads also contain vitamin A (essential for healthy sight and skin) and vitamin D (essential for healthy bones).

Monounsaturated oils, such as olive oil and rapeseed oil, contain small amounts of vitamin

BREAKDOWN OF FATS

Fat	Saturate %	Monoun- saturate %	Polyun- saturate %
Avocado	11	70	13
Butter fat	64	33	3
Coconut	91	7	2
Groundnut	19	45	36
Hazelnut	8	77	11
Olive	14	76	10
Palm	51	39	10
Rapeseed	7	63	30
Safflower	9	14	77
Sesame	14	37	43
Soya bean	15	23	62
Sunflower	11	23	66
Walnut	9	16	70

E, which is needed for the structure of cell walls. Vitamin E is also an antioxidant, which oils require to prevent them from becoming rancid.

Olive oil has become synonymous with healthy eating because it is used in the traditional Mediterranean diet, which has a low incidence of heart disease and cancer. While mono-unsaturates can lower cholesterol, they do not do so as efficiently as polyunsaturates. It's therefore a good idea to use polyunsaturated sunflower or soya oil for cooking and to reserve olive oil, which has the best flavour, for dressings.

Walnut and sesame oils (polyunsaturated) and hazelnut oil (monounsaturated) have distinctive flavours and make delicious dressings, but you might like to temper the flavour by mixing them with bland polyunsaturates, which also makes them go further.

Reduced-fat spreads (containing less than 60 per cent fat) can also be useful in creating a healthy diet. As a rule, choose those in which less than 25 per cent of the fat content is saturated fats. For example, if you use a 60 g per 100 g fat spread, it should not contain more than 15 g of saturated fat per 100 g. Also check the label for trans fat content. If it's not mentioned, the product may contain a lot. Where trans fats are listed, choose spreads with no more than 0.5 g per 100 g.

15. Fish
Eat at least twice a week.

Why should we eat more fish? Oily fish, such as salmon, mackerel, trout, sardines or fresh tuna, is rich in omega-3 fats, which provide us with many health benefits: they make blood less likely to clot, therefore reducing the risk of heart disease and stroke; they improve the elasticity of arteries and help stabilise or prevent harmful irregular heart rhythms. Additionally, their anti-inflammatory properties help to ease chronic health problems affecting the skin and joints.

For many people, eating more fish (oily or white) means eating less meat, thereby lowering the overall intake of harmful saturated fats and replacing them with beneficial fats.

Just two portions of fish a week, at least one being oily fish, will help reduce the risk of heart disease and stroke. Ideally, each of the two weekly servings of fish should provide 200 mg of the omega-3 fats EPA and DHA. As you can see from the table overleaf, an average 160 g/5½ oz portion of mackerel will provide

OMEGA-3 CONTENT OF FISH

Food	Average UK portion	EPA	DPA* g per 100 g food	DHA	Total omega-3 per portion
Cod	120 g	0.08	0.01	0.16	0.30
Cod liver oil	5 ml/1 tsp	10.8	1.40	8.30	1.19
Haddock	120 g	0.05	0.01	0.10	0.19
Herring	119 g	0.51	0.11	0.69	2.18
Mackerel	160 g	0.71	0.12	1.10	4.46
Pilchards, canned in tomato sauce	110 g	1.17	0.23	1.20	3.16
Plaice	130 g	0.16	0.04	0.10	0.42
Prawns, frozen, raw	60 g	0.06	trace	0.04	0.91
Salmon, canned	100 g	0.55	0.14	0.86	1.85
Salmon, fresh	100 g	0.5	0.4	1.3	2.5
Sardines, canned in tomato sauce	100 g	0.89	0.10	0.68	2.02
Trout	230 g	0.23	0.09	0.83	2.92

* This is another type of omega-3 fat, but not widespread or as important as EPA or DHA.

Source: Ω-3 Fatty Acids and Health, British Nutrition Foundation (1999)

more than 4 g of omega-3 fats, so the ideal target is quite achievable. (It also exceeds the UK government recommendation of 1.5 g a week – a good thing.)

Varieties that have edible bones, such as whitebait and canned sardines, also supply calcium. Canned fish generally retain beneficial amounts of their nutritional content, so they are well worth including in your diet, especially since they also retain a lot of their omega-3 content.

Vegetarians who do not eat fish can obtain fatty acids similar to those in oily fish by eating linseeds, walnuts and soya products, but this must be part of a healthy background diet. Some plants contain omega-3 fats, but they are not as effective as those from fish.

White fish, such as cod, haddock, plaice and whiting, are excellent sources of low-fat protein and rich in vitamins B_6 and B_{12}, iron, iodine, selenium and zinc. White fish has a more delicate flavour than oily fish, and the negligible amount of fat it contains is also unsaturated.

As most of us are not in a position to buy fish straight from the nets, the next best option – if you cannot buy fresh from a fishmonger – is to buy fish that has been frozen at sea. Pre-packed fresh fish from the chiller cabinet in the supermarket has been flushed with a mixture of nitrogen, carbon dioxide and oxygen, which slows down bacterial growth and allows it to remain fresh for longer. Fresh fish should, ideally, be eaten on the day of purchase. If the fish has not been previously frozen (which should be stated on the label), it can safely be frozen at home. Thawed fish should not be refrozen.

When buying fish, allow 150 g/5 oz per person for steaks and fillets, and 375 g/13 oz per person for whole fish on the bone. The fishmonger will descale, clean, fillet and skin the fish as you require, if it hasn't already been done. Oily fish are more suited to barbecuing, grilling and baking because they have 'built-in' oils that baste the fish as it cooks. White fish are more delicate, so they are better suited to being steamed and poached.

For optimum health benefits, steam or grill fish, or choose another method of cooking that does not involve adding (saturated) fat. Keep fish and chips and other battered, deep-fried meals for occasional treats.

Easy ways to eat more fish
Use both canned and cold cooked fish to make sandwich fillings in combinations such as salmon and watercress, tuna with chopped pepper or sweetcorn, smoked mackerel with soft cheese and chopped celery.

Top toast with sardines, pilchards or sild (canned herring) in a variety of different sauces, e.g. mustard or tomato.

Make fishcakes using cheaper types of fish, such as coley and mackerel – ideal for mixing with potato and fresh herbs.

Use white and oily fish, shellfish and seafood to make a wide range of curries.

Add freshly cooked fish and shellfish, either hot or cold, to mixed salad leaves.

Combine canned fish with rice and canned vegetables to make quick and tasty meals, e.g. rice, tuna and sweetcorn, or rice, salmon and broad beans. If you're feeling more adventurous, try making paella, a classic combination of rice, fish and shellfish.

16. Yoghurt and probiotics
Eat regularly.

We each have 100 trillion bacteria in our gut, some good, some bad. Eating a healthy diet ensures that the beneficial ones keep the upper hand, and we can assist this by including foods that contain live bacteria, such as yoghurt and probiotic drinks.

To be labelled probiotic (literally 'for life') the bacteria should remain stable and live during the shelf life of the product and withstand the effects of stomach acid and bile during digestion to reach the colon, where they can establish themselves in the gut flora for beneficial effect.

Different friendly bacteria have different benefits: some stimulate the immune system to help fight off harmful bacteria and reduce the duration of food poisoning and stomach upsets; others speed the transit time of waste food through the gut, which helps prevent constipation. On average in the UK, transit time is 40–72 hours: shorter times would be beneficial as waste products are in contact with the gut for a shorter period, reducing the risk of cancer; however, too fast and you end up with diarrhoea.

Friendly bacteria also make anti-adhesives, which help prevent harmful bacteria, and possibly carcinogens, from sticking to the gut. In addition, they neutralise and transport carcinogens out of the body, and produce chemicals that cause cancer cells to 'commit suicide'.

The bacterial colony in the gut needs to be regularly 'topped up' as the beneficial ones are destroyed by antibiotics, food poisoning, stress, poor diet (too much fatty food and not enough NSP), too much alcohol, traveller's diarrhoea, and simply being over 50. Regular intake of yoghurt or other probiotic food and drinks is therefore necessary.

Remember, too, that low-fat yoghurt is an excellent source of calcium, which benefits bone health in all age groups.

SO WHAT ARE PREBIOTICS?
Prebiotics are the 'food' of probiotics – in other words, the substances, such as oligosaccharides and other naturally occurring NSPs, found in vegetables, fruit and whole grains, or added to food during processing. Probiotic bacteria ferment prebiotics to produce protective substances for the immune system and to fight cancer and help lower cholesterol levels.

Easy ways to eat more yoghurt and probiotics
Use instead of milk on breakfast cereal such as granola.

Eat for breakfast with fruit.

Make mayonnaise-style salad dressings with thick natural yoghurt instead of eggs and oil.

Marinate meat, fish and poultry in yoghurt-based marinades (consult your Indian and Oriental recipe books).

Swirl yoghurt on to soups and casseroles as a generous garnish, or stir in to add creaminess without overloading the fat content.

Serve cooling dips, such as raita (yoghurt, cucumber and mint) alongside curries and other spicy dishes.

Eat yoghurt for snacks and desserts.

Serve low-fat yoghurt in place of cream, evaporated milk or condensed milk with desserts.

Make smoothies from puréed fruit mixed with yoghurt.

Drink lassi, an Indian yoghurt-based drink, with meals or as a thirst-quencher at any time.

17. Milk and cheese
Have two or three low-fat portions a day.

Around three-quarters of the calcium in our diet comes from milk, and it also contains B vitamins and a small amount of other minerals, such as zinc, magnesium and phosphorus. The fattier milks contain vitamins A and D, but these are adequately provided in most diets anyway, so there is no need to stop drinking skimmed milks. B vitamins are also present in the non-fat part of the milk, notably B_2 and B_{12}, plus some folates. As B vitamins are light-sensitive, milk bottles should be kept out of the sunlight. Vegetarians who do not consume dairy products can get calcium from oats, muesli, pulses, nuts, dark green vegetables and dried fruit.

Whole or full-fat milk contains about 3.5 per cent fat, semi-skimmed about 1.7 per cent, and skimmed about 1 per cent, so swapping to a low-fat variety can make a useful contribution to lowering your intake of saturated fat, and save you a lot of calories during your lifetime.

Milk and its products are also good sources of protein. Perhaps most popular of these is cheese. Most of Britain's favourite cheeses are high in fat and salt, so they should be eaten in moderation. Remember, a portion is only the size of a matchbox. If using cheese to flavour a dish, choose a mature type because its stronger flavour means that you can use less.

Reduced-fat Cheddar-style cheeses are now available, and while they contain less fat than regular varieties, the mineral content remains the same.

18. Lean red meat and game
Eat in moderation.

Red meat is a good source of iron and zinc, and since many women in the UK lack iron in their diet, eating lean red meat can be a good idea. In general, the redder the meat, the more iron it contains. If possible, buy organic or free-range meat and game as it is likely to be lower in saturated fat than meat from intensively raised livestock that is unable to exercise.

Traditionally, game was a term applied to wild animals, such as deer, pheasant, rabbit, grouse and hare. Nowadays, however, most game is raised for the table, so although some are free-range, they are hardly 'wild'. Game meat is generally lower in fat, particularly saturated fat, than meat from animals reared intensively.

Lean red meat and game are good sources of protein because they contain all the amino acids (building blocks of protein) needed by the body; plant sources do not contain them in the right combinations or amounts.

The iron and zinc in meat are more readily absorbed by the body than those in plant foods. Meat also provides B vitamins, particularly vitamin B_{12}, which is essential for health and not found in plant foods.

A portion of red meat is 80 g/$3\frac{1}{4}$ oz, the equivalent of three smallish slices of beef or steak, three slices of lamb, or two slices of pork. This might be less than many people are used to, but red meat should be eaten in moderation.

In order to keep the fat content of meat and game as low as possible, it is best to stir-fry, casserole, braise or grill it, using sauces (where necessary) that are based on vegetable purées or stock rather than cream. Cook meat thoroughly to avoid food poisoning, but avoid any cooking method that blackens or burns the skin or flesh because the charred parts contain potential carcinogens. If you do eat red meat, you should also eat plenty of vegetables, fruit and wholegrain foods for their anti-cancer properties.

Preserved meat products, such as sausages, bacon and ham, should be avoided or eaten only occasionally because they are high in fat and salt. In addition, there may be a possible connection between as little as 60 g/2¼ oz of processed meat a day and cancer of the bowel and stomach. Remember too that fatty meat products also contribute to weight problems.

VEGETARIAN SOURCES OF IRON AND PROTEIN

Those who do not eat meat or fish can get their protein requirement from pulses, soya products, such as tofu, and Quorn, a myco-protein made from fungi. In a carefully balanced diet, adequate iron can be obtained from whole grains, pulses and vegetables. Note, however, that iron from plant sources is less easily absorbed than iron from animal sources, but it can be improved by including plenty of vitamin C in the diet.

19. Poultry
Eat in moderation.

The term 'poultry' includes all types of domesticated fowl raised for the table. The best known are chicken and turkey, but guinea fowl, duck and geese also fall in this category. The fat content of these birds varies enormously: chicken and turkey are generally the leanest, but even these need to be trimmed of excess fat and the skin should be discarded before serving.

If possible, choose free-range organic birds, as they have a lower fat content and more flavour than those reared intensively. This also applies to corn-fed birds, which are distinguished by having yellowish flesh and fat.

Minced turkey is a useful lower fat alternative to minced beef and lamb, and can be used in just the same ways, such as for making burgers, meatballs and bolognese sauce.

To ensure that the poultry remains low in fat, do not add fat when roasting it. Sit the bird on a trivet (rack) in a roasting pan, breast side down for a third of the cooking time, then invert for the remainder to brown the skin. This method both self-bastes the bird and also allows the fat to drain off into the pan from where it can be discarded before serving the meat, or used to make gravy.

20. Seaweed
Eat as part of the recommended five or more daily portions of fruit and vegetables.

In a traditional Asian diet seaweed is an important food and contributes many minerals, including calcium and iron. It is also an excellent source of iodine and selenium, which are needed for the production of thyroid hormones that control the metabolic rate (see page 97). In a Western diet sea fish and shellfish are the main sources of these two minerals, but they are also found in vegetables, fruit and cereals. The other minerals in seaweed include manganese and copper, plus small amounts of molybdenum, cobalt and chromium.

Seaweed's fat content (less than 1 per cent) is rich in omega-3 fats. It is also high in fibre and

ADD FLAVOUR WITHOUT SALT

It takes time to become accustomed to eating food without salt, but the health benefits are so great that it's worth making the effort.

The best way to give extra flavour to food is by adding herbs and spices. As every culture in the world has combinations that are specific to its cuisine, there is ample opportunity to experiment and bring new interest to your own cooking.

Bouquet garni, for example, is a French herb combination consisting usually of a few sprigs of parsley, a sprig of thyme and one or two dried bay leaves. (In some regions it can include rosemary, bay, basil and savory.) Whatever the content, the herbs are tied together and simmered in stocks or sauces to impart their aromatic flavours. By contrast, the most common combination of herbs in Thai cooking is flatleaf parsley, coriander, kaffir lime leaves and lemon grass. The resulting flavour could not be more different from bouquet garni, but it is equally aromatic and delicious. Let these classic examples inspire you to experiment with herbs to flavour your own cooking.

When buying herbs, choose those with healthy-looking and lush green growth. Pots of herbs, such as parsley, basil, coriander, chives, dill and thyme, should be watered sparingly because over-watering dilutes their flavour.

Another way to add flavour in the absence of salt is to use spices, such as black pepper, cloves, cumin, ginger, saffron and turmeric. These may be available in different forms – fresh, dried, ground or preserved. Ready-made spice mixtures, such as Cajun seasoning, Chinese five-spice powder and garam masala, can also be very useful. And don't forget spice pastes, such as fiery harissa from north Africa and Thai curry pastes, which can be used to add heat and flavour to fish, meat and their vegetarian substitutes.

contains antioxidants, which protect against heart disease.

Various parts of the UK have a tradition of incorporating seaweed into the diet: the Welsh boil and mash laver to make laverbread, while the Scots use dulse as a vegetable and add it to soups. Far Eastern cuisines make more inspirational use of seaweeds, particularly kombu, nori and wakame. These are wrapped around rice, fish and vegetables to make sushi.

For seaweed to make any nutritional contribution to your diet, you would have to eat it regularly and in quantity.

Easy ways to eat more seaweed
Use sheets of kombu, nori and wakame (available from specialist food shops) in

KEEP HYDRATED AND HEALTHY

Now you have all the information you need to create a healthy diet, don't forget that you need to drink 1.5–2 litres/2½–3½ pints of liquid per day, the equivalent of about eight to 10 drinks, if each one is about 200 ml/7 fl oz. Ideally, your drinks should include lots of water. (Some people find it useful to have a 1 litre bottle that they refill as necessary so that they can keep track of how much they have drunk.)

Plain water is the best drink for quenching thirst, but you can flavour the occasional glass with low-sugar squash or cordial if you like. However, it's not good for teeth or waistline to sip sugary drinks all day.

Fruit juice and skimmed milk can also make up one or two of the drinks each day. Fruit juice may be diluted to reduce its acid effects on the teeth, but if you drink only one or two glasses a day, it is not a problem. Alcohol does not count at all towards your fluid intake.

Although it's fine to drink some tea and coffee, don't have all your intake in these forms. Tea and coffee are diuretics, which means they cause increased urination and the loss of water-soluble vitamins. Their caffeine content can also be over-stimulating. Perhaps try herb and fruit teas instead.

It must be noted, however, that regular tea drinkers seem to have a reduced risk of heart disease. Just one cup a day seems to benefit both men and women, and the benefits increase by drinking up to four. After that, you are probably overdoing it. The benefits in tea come from the antioxidants quercetin and catechin, which help to neutralise free radicals and thus prevent hardening of the arteries – a risk for heart attacks and stroke.

Black tea, the type most popular in the UK, also contains fluoride, which protects teeth from the acid-producing bacteria in dental plaque. Green tea also helps to slow and repair tooth decay, but, even more impressively, laboratory experiments have shown that the catechin in green tea inhibits the growth of cancer cells.

salads, stir-fries, stocks and soups, or crumbled on to food as a condiment in place of salt.

Buy ready-made sushi lunchboxes instead of sandwiches for a change.

Try eating out in Japanese restaurants where more 'gourmet' but healthy seaweed dishes appear on the menu.

Drink kombu tea.

Chapter 4

Be more active

There's no denying it – your activity level is as important as the amount you eat when it comes to controlling weight and preventing chronic diseases.

Having read this far, you will be familiar with the fact that 'calories in' have to equal 'calories out' in order to prevent weight gain. In other words, if the number of calories you eat is consistently greater than the number you use up, you will put on weight.

Until recently there was a tendency to take a rather simplistic view of managing weight problems, namely, eat less and you'll get thinner. But when nutrition experts observed that people were eating less but that obesity and weight problems were rising, they realised something else must be going on.

When you stop to think about it, the explanation is obvious: we are not active enough. People are putting on weight, even though eating less, because activity levels have declined even faster than our food intake. It doesn't take a genius to observe that motorised transport, escalators, labour-saving equipment, Internet shopping and remote control devices are doing the hard physical work for us. We spend increasing amounts of time in front of computer and television screens instead of doing something physical. Of course, you know all this.

The bottom line is that sloth may be as important as gluttony in creating the problem of excess weight.

DIETING MAKES IT WORSE

When people put on weight few of them think, 'Yippee! I'll become more active.' Instead the usual reaction is, 'Oh no, I'll have to go on a diet – again.' But diets can make matters worse.

When you drastically reduce your intake on a low-calorie diet your body goes into starvation mode and decreases the rate at which you burn calories. Alongside this lower metabolic rate (explained on page 97–8), your body also tends (particularly without exercise) to lose lean tissue (muscle) rather than fat. Less lean tissue means you need fewer calories because muscle burns energy, fat doesn't.

The legacy of going on a very low-calorie diet is that as soon as you return to your previous eating habits (and you will), you simply put on fat more quickly and become even heavier than before. That's why gradual but permanent diet and lifestyle change is the only way to control weight once and for all.

EXERCISING MAKES IT BETTER

It takes one hour of moderate to intense activity, such as walking, on most days of the week to maintain a healthy body weight. This is particularly the case for people with sedentary occupations.

We'd all be a lot less prone to weight problems and chronic disease if we were more active.

HOW MUCH EXERCISE IS NEEDED TO PREVENT CHRONIC DISEASE?

The risk for all chronic diseases reduces with increased activity levels. As stated above, the ideal amount for weight control is one hour a day, yet it does not take that much to reduce the risk of some other health problems.

Heart disease: At least 30 minutes of moderate to intense physical activity each day is enough to improve cardiovascular function to protect against heart disease.
Warning: People who do not take regular exercise, or who have a high risk of heart disease, should avoid sudden bursts of high-intensity exercise, such as squash.

Type 2 diabetes: Preventive measures include an endurance activity at a moderate (or higher) level of intensity, e.g. brisk walking, for one hour or more a day on most days of the week. This takes into account that prevention or treatment of excess weight is necessary to reduce the risk of type 2 diabetes, and that reducing or preventing abdominal obesity is also a major goal in preventing it.

Cancer: Vigorous activity, such as fast walking, may give benefits for preventing some cancers, such as cancer of the colon. As obesity is a major risk factor in cancer, as much as one hour may be needed, as for weight control (see above).

Osteoporosis: Prevention requires a lifetime of weight-bearing activity. In youth, vigorous weight-bearing activity that includes impact on bones is needed to increase peak bone mass. This helps maintain bone mass in later life, when activities that maintain or increase muscle strength, and that encourage coordination and balance, help prevent falls that lead to osteoporotic fractures.

While making this one hour a day recommendation in their 2003 report, the WHO recognises that it differs from national governments' advice, including the UK's, that 30 minutes of moderate activity on most days is adequate. Although agreeing that people of all ages would be healthier if they managed even 30 minutes, the WHO experts say it probably takes one hour's activity on most days for sedentary people (specifically) to control their weight.

Although one hour might seem an impossible target, remember that the daily total can be broken down into several short bouts, making it more feasible, and that household chores and normal activities also 'count'. For example, an hour's exercise could be made up of two brisk 20-minute walks (perhaps accompanying the children to and from school, doing a paper round or distributing leaflets), plus 10 minutes climbing stairs and 10 minutes cleaning the kitchen floor. Yet in the UK only one quarter of men and women meet the recommendation of at least 30 minutes of moderate to vigorous aerobic activity on five or more occasions per week.

IT'S ALL GOOD STUFF

Any amount of regular physical activity is good for you. The amount or frequency is more important than the intensity. For example, being moderately active on a daily basis may take longer to lower your cholesterol than jogging 30 km/19 miles a week, but it will do so just as effectively, eventually. And even if you lose only a little weight, activity will improve your health in many other respects. It will:

- Maximise loss of fat.
- Increase muscle, which improves your body tone and shape (the aim of most dieters) and can help with weight loss if sustained.
- Stimulate your metabolic rate to burn more calories.
- Build healthier bones because weight-bearing exercise (walking, skipping, even shopping) stimulates bone mineralisation.
- Improve your mood and fight mild depression by boosting production of endorphins, nature's feel-good hormones.
- Reduce stress by releasing feel-good endorphins. And since many people find comfort in food when feeling stressed, this also helps reduce food intake.
- Lower your total cholesterol level and increase the ratio of good to bad (HDL to LDL) cholesterol.
- Protect your health by lowering the risk of all those chronic diseases discussed in Chapters 1 and 2.

WHAT'S STOPPING YOU?

Two of the biggest barriers to taking enough exercise are not having the time, and the myth that exercise has to hurt to be beneficial.

While you can't add more hours to your day, you can become more active in the hours you have. And you can find ways to enjoy physical activity as part of your life. It does not have to be something divorced from day-to-day activity: it can include walking or cycling to the shops, brisk housework and gardening, cleaning cars and windows, playing with your children in the park... (For more ideas see opposite.)

Lots of healthy lifestyle leaflets encourage more activity as part of your life. When they suggest that you 'walk or cycle some or all of the way to work', 'take the stairs', or 'go for a walk in your lunch hour' have you ever wondered what the pay-off is for being more active? How many calories do those activities use?

Check it out opposite, then try to incorporate as many of those activities as you can into your day-to-day life. They will help you lose weight, tone up and even have fun while you acquire a more active outlook.

BURNING CALORIES

You don't have to go to the gym to get fit: there are lots of ways to incorporate more exercise into your life, whether you are home-based, out at work or just on the move. All calorie counts given for the activities opposite are calculated for the average UK woman aged 35 who weighs 70 kg/11 stone. If you

WHAT'S IT WORTH?

ACTIVITY (duration per day, unless stated otherwise)	CALORIES

On the move

• Run for the bus (200 metres/200 yards)	15
• Get off the bus one stop early (400 metres/440 yards)	25
• Climb stairs rather than take lifts (15 minutes)	100
• Play in a swimming pool with the kids (15 minutes)	100
• Play Frisbee in the park (30 minutes)	100
• Cycle to work or school at 14 kph/9 mph (30 minutes)	150
• Walk to the shops pushing a buggy, pram or shopping trolley (15 minutes each way)	200
• Swim at a moderate speed (20 minutes)	200
• Walk at a moderate pace of 5 kph/3 mph (60 minutes)	250
• Walk briskly at 7 kph/4.5 mph (60 minutes)	300
• Slow jog at 10 kph/6 mph (60 minutes)	100
• Flex your ankles and feet while sitting at your desk (once an hour for five minutes over five eight-hour days)	500
• Kick boxing (60 minutes)	700

At home

Whether you are at home all the time or just at weekends, there are lots of small changes you can make to burn more calories and lose weight. Women with small children will find this particularly helpful as weight often increases when activity levels drop after giving up outside work.

• Clean your teeth with a manual toothbrush instead of an electric one (twice a day, seven days a week)	56
• Clean windows (30 minutes)	100
• Do buttock clenches or squats while working at the kitchen counter: pretend to sit on a chair, clenching your buttocks just before you would sit down (three minutes per day over five days)	100
• Shovel snow from paths or driveway (10 minutes)	100
• March around, military style, keeping pace to fast music (15 minutes a day)	100
• Scrub the kitchen floor on hands and knees instead of using a mop	100–200
• Play tennis, ping-pong or badminton (30 minutes)	200
• Wash and polish the car	300
• Lie on the floor and do side leg lifts as you listen to a child reading, or while watching TV (10 minutes, seven nights a week)	300
• Decorate a room (60 minutes)	300
• Garden more energetically than gentle weeding (60 minutes)	350
• Spring-clean a room (two hours)	400
• Re-organise the furniture in a room (60 minutes)	400
• Do low-impact aerobics (60 minutes)	400
• Do high-impact aerobics, such as BodyPump, Body Combat or Step (60 minutes)	500
• Fidget: in an average day a fidget can burn off much more energy than a non-fidget	500

are heavier, you will burn a few more calories; if you are lighter, you will burn slightly fewer. But remember: doing more physical activity is not only about calories and weight loss; it is also about improving general health.

WHAT AM I AIMING FOR?

The aim of taking more exercise is to be as physically active as someone with an active occupation, such as a gardener, builder or farmer. Our ancestors were certainly a lot more active than we are, and our bodies are built to function at a higher level of activity than our sedentary jobs and home lives provide. If the suggestions in the table below do not appeal or are impractical for you, aim to walk briskly for 30 minutes to one hour a day, and also do at least one hour a week of activity at a higher intensity, such as a sport or dancing.

BUSY DOING NOTHING

Get into the habit of relaxing and doing 'nothing' in a more energetic way and you will be surprised how slimming it can be.

ACTIVITY	CALORIES
• Have energetic sex (30 minutes)	50
• Have gentle sex (30 minutes)	30
• Do Pilates or yoga (40 minutes)	100
• Do sit-ups as you watch TV (10 minutes)	100
• Play the piano (30 minutes)	100
• Walk up and down stairs while using a cordless phone (30 minutes)	100
• Try line dancing (30 minutes)	100
• Abandon the remote control and walk to the TV (three times a day over a year)	200
• Go salsa dancing (30 minutes)	200

HOW CAN BEING MORE ACTIVE PREVENT CANCER?

We are all familiar with the evidence that exercise can help weight control and improve fitness by training the heart and lungs to work more efficiently. However, the link between activity and cancer prevention is less obvious. You can feel the effect of exercise on your heart and lungs (your heart beats faster and you become breathless), but you cannot see what's going on inside your body at a cellular level as a result of physical activity.

Nonetheless, it is known that the more active you are, the lower your risk of certain cancers. For example, physically active men and women halve their risk of developing bowel cancer, and there may also be benefits for breast cancer and other cancers. This is possibly because of the favourable effect of exercise on insulin levels and sex hormones, which both influence cell growth and division. (Cancer occurs when cell division goes wrong.)

In the case of bowel cancer, the other beneficial effect of exercise is to speed 'bowel transit time' – the time it takes for food and food waste to travel through the gut. Faster transit means that potential carcinogens are in contact with the lining of the colon for less time.

EXCESS WEIGHT AND CANCER

A lot of people are puzzled by this connection. How can being obese make you 25–30 per cent more likely to get colon cancer, prostate cancer, endometrial cancer, oesophageal cancer, kidney cancer and post-menopausal breast cancer?

When you have a lot of body fat, the body makes more sex hormones. Fat is a site for sex hormone synthesis in men, and particularly in post-menopausal women (a time of life when cancer rates rise). Sex hormones influence cell division in sites such as the breast, endometrium and prostate. The higher the level of sex hormones, the more sites they can bind to, within which they can potentially create cell division that may turn into cancer.

Breast and endometrial cancer in women and prostate cancer in men are usually sex hormone-related cancers, so being overweight is a risk factor in developing them. Athletes have lower levels of circulating testosterone, showing that exercise can lower levels of this hormone, which is known to influence development of prostate cancer. Physical activity also changes the way sex hormones are used by the body, providing a protective effect.

Overweight bodies tend to develop an unhealthy relationship with insulin. The more fat they contain, the more insulin is made, and the more likely it is that insulin resistance will develop. If it does develop, insulin production is further increased to try to compensate for the resistance. The more insulin there is, the more potential there is for things to go wrong. That's because when cells receive insulin, they get more blood sugar and they divide, and when cells divide, there are more chances for that process to go wrong and a tumour to occur.

Higher levels of insulin also inhibit a natural process called apoptosis (cell suicide), which prevents potentially carcinogenic cells from self-destructing. This means that cancer cells can reproduce themselves unchecked and lead to more serious problems.

WHAT SHOULD I DO TO REDUCE MY CANCER RISK IF I AM TOO FAT?

When the American Institute of Cancer Research (AICR) pronounced in 2002 on the link between being fat and having a higher risk of cancer, it advised people to do more than simply lose weight. It advocated a low-fat diet rich in fruits, vegetables, whole grains and beans because they contain nutrients that fight cancer; it recommended keeping weight gain during adulthood to a maximum of 5 kg/11 lb (in line with WHO recommendations); and it suggested taking one hour of moderate exercise a day, plus one hour of vigorous exercise a week to help lose weight, modulate insulin release and speed the expulsion of toxins from the body.

The last suggestion might sound a bit 'alternative', especially given the currently fashionable pastime of detoxing, but the AICR explains that fat traps carcinogens (from food, the air and other sources), so physical activity is important to burn off fat.

An article published in *Lancet Oncology*, the UK's leading medical cancer journal, in 2002 concludes that you have the lowest risk of developing cancer if you have a body mass index (BMI) of 18.5–25 (see page 18), so long as you do not have a lot of body fat within that BMI range. For more about the proportion of fat to body weight, see page 89.

Lancet Oncology also advises: 'The best way to achieve a healthy body weight is to balance energy intake with energy expenditure. Excess body fat can be reduced by restricting calorific intake and increasing physical activity. Calorific intake can be reduced by decreasing the size of food portions and limiting the intake of

NATIONAL GAME PLAN

The Strategy Unit at 10 Downing Street issued a report on the nation's health in December 2002. *Game Plan*, as it was called, sets a goal for a massive increase in the number of people who exercise regularly or take part in sport. Currently, around 30 per cent of the UK population is 'reasonably active' (about 30 minutes five times a week), although not all polls and surveys support this figure. However, as physical inactivity contributes to 54,000 premature deaths a year in the UK at a cost of £2 billion, *Game Plan* wants to see 70 per cent of the population taking regular exercise by 2020.

calorie-dense foods that are high in fat and refined sugars. Such foods should be replaced with foods like vegetables, fruits, whole grains and beans.'

Far more difficult to prove scientifically, but confirmed by observation and common sense,

Inactivity may be as bad for the heart as smoking 20 cigarettes a day because it doubles the chance of heart disease, raises the risk of blood pressure by one third and type 2 diabetes by a half.

World Health Federation report for World Heart Day, September 2002 is that people who exercise tend to eat a better diet and use less alcohol and tobacco, which also reduces their risk of cancer.

So what are you waiting for? Alter your ratio of fat to muscle, and you'll burn more calories and look sexier.

MONITOR YOUR BODY FAT

It could be argued that your health, specifically avoiding heart disease, diabetes and certain cancers, depends less on how much you weigh and more on what proportion of your weight is body fat. This surprising revelation means that on the outside someone might look great and even be an 'ideal' clothes size, but they could have a high proportion of body fat and therefore be at far greater risk than their stocky and physically fit best friend whose body contains a higher proportion of muscle. (Note that muscle weighs heavier than fat.)

Standard bathroom scales tell you only one side of the story. They cannot give you your body composition, but body-fat monitor scales can. You feed in information about your weight, height and age, then you stand barefoot on the machine and an electrical current is passed painlessly through your body. Instead of displaying your weight, the machine tells you what percentage of your body is fat.

This information may be even more useful than knowing your body mass index (see page 18) because two people can have the same BMI, but the one with higher body-fat composition has greater health risks.

Your body shape, genetic make-up – whether you put on weight around the waist (bad news), at the hips and bum (not such bad news), and whether you are naturally muscular or prone to laying down internal fat – will all determine your percentage of body fat. Age comes into it too because we all carry more fat as we get older. Ethnicity also plays a part: Asians from the Indian subcontinent have the highest fat mass for their BMI, and black Africans the lowest; Caucasians, followed by the Japanese, fall between these two groups. Only 2.6 per cent of Japanese women and 1.8 per cent of men are obese compared with 21 per cent of UK women and 17 per cent of men.

WHAT SHOULD YOUR BODY-FAT PERCENTAGE BE?

As yet there is no agreed international standard for body-fat percentages. However, leading researchers in the field have come up with a range of healthy body-fat percentages based on World Health Organisation BMIs, as listed below.

Sex/Age	Healthy	Overfat	Obese
	body-fat percentage		
Women 20–39	21–33	34–38	39+
Women 40–59	23–34	35–40	41+
Women 60–79	24–36	37–42	43+
Men 20–39	8–20	21–25	26+
Men 40–59	11–22	23–28	29+
Men 60–79	13–25	26–30	31+

It is also unhealthy not to have enough fat. Young women who are too thin are at risk of anaemia, and too little calcium can result in osteoporosis later in life. Amenorrhoea (missing menstrual periods) is common in women with not enough fat, and can lead to infertility.

Some body-fat monitors also give a total body-water reading. This is useful because good water levels in the body are essential for physical and mental performance. Again, there are no agreed international levels, but healthy women should have total water readings of 50–55 per cent and men 60–65 per cent.

TOO BUSY TO LIVE LONGER

Fewer than a quarter of UK women are exercising enough to protect their health, says

STRETCH THOSE ARTERIES

Exercise of any sort also helps prevent arteries stiffening, which they do with age and inactivity. People who build exercise into their daily routine have stretchier arteries, and those who have been active throughout their life have the stretchiest arteries into their 80s and 90s. They also tend to have lower blood-sugar levels, another bonus as raised blood sugar and excess insulin can also stiffen arteries.

Hardening of the arteries is a separate and additional risk to blocked arteries. As mentioned earlier, physical activity contributes to lower cholesterol levels and to a healthier ratio of good to bad cholesterol. And, as you know, lower cholesterol levels reduce the risk of blocked arteries. Yet another good reason to get active.

the organisation Cancer Research UK. And the reasons those women give are lack of time and motivation.

According to the British Heart Foundation (BHF), two out of five deaths from heart disease among women are also due to lack of exercise. Inactive pastimes and coping with stress by passive activities, such as watching television, smoking, drinking alcohol and snacking on comfort foods, are to blame, say the BHF. Some women may consider that rushing around all day is activity enough, but walking and cycling or other forms of exercise for about two and half hours a week, or five 30-minute sessions, would really make a difference – and help reduce stress, too.

'But I never get five minutes to myself,' many women cry. This is rarely the case, even though it might feel like that. However, if 30-minute sessions are a problem, split them up into smaller units that can be fitted around other commitments. The best way to do this is by 'active living', which incorporates moderate exercise into daily activities. There are many opportunities for this, as shown in the list below.

ACTIVE LIVING
- Washing and waxing a car for 45–60 minutes
- Washing windows or floors for 45–60 minutes
- Playing football or a similar game for 45 minutes
- Gardening for 30–45 minutes
- Walking 2.8 km/1¾ miles in 35 minutes (a 20-minute mile)

MAXIMUM HEART RATE

To exercise safely you should not exceed your maximum heart rate (MHR), which is the maximum rate at which your heart beats. The rough rule of thumb in determining your maximum heart rate is 220 beats per minute minus your age. So if you are 40 years old, your MHR would be 220 – 40 = 180 beats per minute.

You can measure your heart rate by taking your pulse at your neck or wrist: rest the fingertip of your second finger on the pulse and count against a second hand on a clock or watch. Alternatively, use a heart-rate monitor, which straps around your chest and transmits information to a device fastened around the wrist. (Using a monitor removes the need to stop and take your pulse while you work out.)

To burn fat you need to work at around 65–75 per cent of your MHR, and to increase cardiovascular fitness you must work at 80–85 per cent of your MHR.

Taking the example above of 180 beats per minute, 85 per cent = 0.85 x 180, which is 153. This is fine if you are otherwise fit and healthy and have no heart or general health problems that might lead you, or your doctor, to believe it is unsafe for you to do aerobic exercise.

There are two basic ways to use MHR. The first is to gradually raise your heart rate during your warm-up to the level at which you want to work and maintain it for 25 minutes (less if you are not yet fit). Then slow down to lower your heart rate back to normal during your warm-down. Alternatively, practise 'interval training', where you work to a lower MHR during your warm-up (around 60–65 per cent). Keep this as the base rate throughout your 25 minutes of core activity, but include four or more two-minute bursts at a harder rate to rise to around 80 per cent MHR. Following each burst, return to the base rate for four or five minutes. Warm down in the usual way.

- Propelling yourself in a wheelchair for 30–40 minutes
- Playing basketball or volleyball for 15–20 minutes
- Shooting baskets for 30 minutes
- Pushing a pram or buggy 2.5 km/1½ miles in 30 minutes (a 20-minute mile)
- Cycling 8 km/5 miles in 30 minutes
- Raking leaves for 30 minutes
- Walking 3 km/2 miles in 30 minutes (a 15-minute mile)

- Dancing fast for 30 minutes
- Water aerobics for 30 minutes
- Shovelling snow for 15 minutes
- Swimming lengths for 20 minutes
- Climbing stairs or using a step machine for 15 minutes
- Cycling 5.4 km/4 miles in 15 minutes
- Skipping for 15 minutes
- Running 2.5 km/1½ miles in 15 minutes (a 10-minute mile)

Inspired to become more active?

If you are aiming to start doing five or more 30-minute activity sessions a week and you have not done any or much activity for some time, it is important to build up slowly over a period of weeks. Depending where you are starting from, this might mean exercising five minutes a day to start with, and building up in five-minute increments each week until you can manage the full 30 minutes. If in doubt, talk to your GP or ask a practice nurse for advice before starting.

WARM UP AND WARM DOWN

All exercise routines should start with a gentle warm-up of around 10 minutes to raise the core temperature of the working muscles, and end with a warm-down of around five minutes to stretch the muscles and prevent a build-up of lactic acid, which can result in post-exercise soreness. The final stretch is not a cool-down (as it is sometimes called) because you want to keep the muscles warm; if you don't, injuries are more likely to occur.

Three simple stretches

1. To stretch the hamstring, stand with feet together facing forwards. Bend one leg at the knee and extend the other leg out straight in front of you, resting the heel on the ground with the foot flexed and the toes pointing upwards. Lean forward slightly, with your hands resting lightly on your thighs, but keep your head and chest raised, and your hips facing forward and aligned. You should feel a stretch in the hamstring of the out-stretched leg. Hold for around 30 seconds, then repeat for the other leg.

2. To stretch the front of the thigh, stand on one leg, holding a wall for support with one hand. With other other hand, reach behind you and carefully raise the other foot by holding the front of the ankle. Gently pull the foot towards the buttock with the knees together to feel a stretch down the front of the thigh. Hold for 30 seconds, then repeat with the other leg.

3. To stretch the calf, stand on a step or a book with the heels overhanging the edge, then gently lower the heels so that you feel a stretch in the calf muscles. Hold for 30 seconds, then repeat if you want.

Note: New research shows that there is no benefit in stretching after the initial warm-up before you go into your walk, jog or run. It was once thought that doing so reduced the risk of injury, but the warm-up itself has been proved sufficient.

Three types of exercise

1. Aerobic or cardiovascular exercise strengthens the heart and improves the body's ability to extract oxygen from the blood and transport it around the body. It also helps you to burn fat for weight reduction. Activities such as walking, jogging, swimming and using fitness equipment for rowing, running, stepping and cross-training fall under this category.

2. Strength or resistance training makes muscles stronger, and also strengthens bones and joints. The resistance comes from working with weights and weight-machines, or against your own body, as in

press-ups, lunges and squats. Building more muscle means that you have the potential to burn more fat.

3. **Stretching and flexing**, as in yoga and Pilates, lengthen muscles (as opposed to building bulk) because they improve strength. They also incorporate breathing techniques and body awareness, which help with stress reduction and relaxation.

Which exercise should you choose?

The following text discusses several of the most widely available and popular exercise options to help you choose what might suit you. But this is not a fitness manual, so you will need either to consult a fitness instructor or buy a good book on the subject for more detailed advice about your chosen activities.

Perhaps the best option for increasing activity is actually the easiest. It requires no classes, no special equipment and no one need know why you're doing it…

Walking

Whether you have had a triple heart bypass or have nothing wrong with you but just don't want to be a couch potato, then walking is the ideal exercise.

Warm-up – start your session by walking at a slowish pace for five to eight minutes to increase circulation and breathing. The speed you continue at determines how many calories per minute you burn and the degree to which your fitness will improve.

The table shows that the heavier you are, the more calories you will burn because of the extra work involved in moving a larger mass.

Core time – walk at the pace you enjoy. Most people find 5.6 kph/3.5 mph comfortable, which translates to a 17-minute mile. Walking at that pace regularly for quite a while will burn fat in a comfortable way. Walkers are more successful at losing weight if they walk longer distances at comfortable speeds. Going all out at a demanding pace simply makes them give up. The paces suggested below burn off fat but are not intense enough to have a training effect.

To achieve cardiovascular fitness (healthy heart and lungs) you must train at a higher intensity, so a brisker walk is needed. You need to work at a higher percentage of your maximum heart rate (MHR, see page 91) so that you will be more breathless and sweatier.

To combine weight loss and cardiovascular conditioning push yourself harder on alternate days so that you have one higher intensity day of brisk walking or jogging, followed by a lower intensity day of moderate walking.

Walking speed		Weight		
	44 kg/7 st	66 kg/10½ st		88 kg/14 st
4.8 kph/3 mph	2.8 cals	4.2 cals		5.6 cals
5.6 kph/3.5 mph	3.3 cals	5.0 cals		6.7 cals
6.4 kph/4 mph	3.8 cals	5.7 cals		7.6 cals

As you continue to walk, you will find you can walk further without your muscles being so sore. Gradually increasing your mileage will have benefits for muscles and fitness. By week six you could be walking 19 km/12 miles a week. Within six weeks you could have progressed to 32 km/20 miles a week.

The reward for increasing the pace to become fitter is a lower risk of developing heart disease. If you are a regular walker who also does some vigorous exercise, you will lower your risk of heart disease even further.

Warm-down – always slow down gradually for five to ten minutes rather than stopping abruptly, and stretch afterwards to prevent soreness.

Jogging and running

If you like the independence of exercising when you choose, rather than according to gym opening hours or class times, and want something more demanding than walking, you simply need to increase the pace and start jogging. You can do this alone, with a friend, or even join a local jogging or running club.

Warm-up – set off at a brisk walking pace for about five minutes, swinging your arms vigorously to get the blood circulating and increase the rate of breathing.

Core time – gradually start on a slow jog and go at a pace that allows you to hold a conversation. If you are too breathless to speak, slow down or walk until you recover, then set off again.

At your first attempt try 10 minutes divided between jogging and walking, and the next day take a walk only. On the third day do a run/walk for 10 minutes again. Gradually reduce the walking part and increase the jogging time on your alternate jogging days.

Then, when you are comfortable at that level, increase the distance or time slightly on every third jog until you are managing 30 minutes three times a week (or fewer if you are doing different activities on the other 'jogging' days).

Warm-down – slow down gradually after each jog until you are walking and your heart rate and breathing are back to normal. It won't take long for you to recognise a return to normality, but if you want a more accurate indication, you could take your pulse (see page 000). While you are still warm, stretch out your muscles.

BUILDING UP THE BENEFIT

As you get fitter, it is important to alter your speed and distance because the body can become accustomed to the same routine, eventually making less effort and therefore burning fewer calories to do it and not improving your fitness. Make it a habit to change your pace: for example, alternate running hard for one minute with jogging for one minute, or, if you are on a track, measure the changes in 200-metre units; if on the street or in the park, mark out the units between certain lampposts or trees.

If you find having a goal or a challenge useful for motivation, you might consider entering a 'race' a few months after you have got used to jogging or running. You could build up to a distance of 5 km/3 miles, train for six weeks at least, and make sure you can run further than the distance of the race.

Joining a gym

Another option for increasing physical activity is to join a gym. Before you do so, it is wise to check out a few things. There are industry associations and registers of exercise professionals, so check the status of the club and its trainers. Make sure the facilities and activities match what you need. For example, if you want to swim, ensure that there is a pool; if you have young children, check that a crêche is available. Are there classes to suit your preferences? Are there outdoor facilities for tennis and badminton? Can you get a membership discount for using the club outside peak hours? Will you have to pay extra for classes or activities, or to use saunas, towels and lockers? Does membership entitle you to use other clubs owned by a chain? Are there spa or beauty treatments available so that you can relax or reward yourself for your efforts? Can you get massage, physiotherapy or osteopathy treatments?

Ensure you have a proper one-to-one induction with an instructor who draws up a personal plan for you after assessing your fitness, taking a medical history and finding out what you want to achieve. He or she should also show you how to use the equipment safely. Don't forget to ask if there is a follow-up session to monitor your progress.

Some clubs have a free trial period, from a day to a week. And each July the UK government backs a Commit to Get Fit campaign. Participating clubs offer short-term memberships so that you can see if a club is right for you. Charity fund-raising events are linked to the campaign. For example, Cancer Research UK organises sponsored 5-km/3-mile runs around the country, under the banner 'Race for Life', to raise money for breast cancer research. Contact your preferred charities or local authority to see if they organise such events.

Before you commit to gym membership, you might like to log on to the Department of Fair Trading's website (www.oft.gov.uk), which has an article called 'Are they fit to join?', which examines the terms and conditions in fitness club contracts.

INITIAL ASSESSMENT

Before your initial assessment with an instructor (you can choose whether to have a male or female for this), think about your aims. What is your main reason for going to the gym? Weight loss? Increased fitness to improve health and prevent chronic disease? Greater strength? Flatter stomach? More flexibility? Better muscle tone? Improved core strength, stability and balance? Perhaps you want all those things. The instructor will ask you about these in order to work out your exercise programme.

The exercise programme will include a warm-up and warm-down, and the activities will depend on what you wish to achieve. They are likely to include an aerobic activity, such as using a treadmill or exercise bike, to gently raise your heart rate. This might be followed by using other gym equipment to tone major muscle groups, then perhaps another bout of aerobic activity, such as rowing, before finishing with stretches. Make a note in your diary to review your progress with an instructor who can update the programme to suit your progress and needs.

Alongside the gym workouts, you need a calorie-controlled or healthy diet, such as one of those outlined in Chapter 5, to ensure you reach your weight loss goals and to fuel your fitness. You'll want some healthy snacks to keep you going, and lots of water – 1 litre/ 2 pints for every hour's training you do (tea and coffee don't count). This is in addition to the 1.5 litres/2½ pints a day recommended for everyone. If you regularly take lots of exercise, aim to consume about 2–2.5 litres/3½–4½ pints of water a day.

Working out with weights

Exercising with weights is a form of resistance training that strengthens muscles. You can work with free (hand-held) weights or weighted gym machines, work against your own body weight (e.g. press-ups and chin-lifts), or take a class, such as BodyPump, that incorporates lifting weights. Whatever you opt for, the idea is to combine high-repetition weight training with aerobic conditioning.

A class involves a warm-up using light weights, and runs through all the major muscle groups (shoulders, biceps, triceps, quadriceps or thighs, and back) to raise the core temperature of the muscles. This is followed by specific exercises for each set of muscles, floor exercises for abdominals, then a warm-down stretch. The aim is to strengthen muscles rather than build bulk. If you don't have access to this type of class, find a good video or book that shows how to work with hand weights at home, or ask an instructor at a gym.

Swimming

You will gain most benefit from swimming if you are proficient in two different strokes, but don't be put off if you are not at that level. Consider taking classes to improve your technique, then aim to swim one to three times a week for about 30 minutes at a time. After six weeks, you will see significant improvements. If you want to increase your fitness levels and swimming is your only activity, you will need to go at least three times a week.

The basic swimming session below covers a total of 800 m/½ mile, once you have reached the greatest number of lengths.

Warm-up – swim 6–12 lengths of 25 metres at a comfortable pace, with a 20–30 second rest after each length. Use two strokes if you can, alternating them for each length.

Core time – swim 5–7 lengths of 50 metres (two 25-metre lengths without stopping) with a 30–40 second rest between each 50 metres.

Warm-down – swim 4–6 lengths of 25 metres at an easy pace. Alternatively, ask the swimming coach at your local pool for some swimming drills, or join a local swimming club.

After you have ben swimming the 800-metre distance for a week or more, *gradually* increase the core-time distance to 900 m/ 1000 yards for a week or two, then increase to 1000 m/1100 yards and so on.

IRON – ESSENTIAL FOR EXERCISE

The mineral iron is used to make haemoglobin, the part of the red blood cell that carries oxygen from the lungs to every part of the body to produce energy. Iron is used in the energy production process itself, so a diet that lacks iron can lead to tiredness and anaemia.

Dwindling iron stores are thought to affect one in three British women of child-bearing age. Studies show that non-physically fit women who are iron deficient (but not bad enough to be anaemic or know they have a problem) attain better levels of fitness if their iron intake is increased. For more information about how to meet your daily requirement of iron, see page 166.

Foods rich in iron include lean red meat, liver, shellfish, oily fish, fortified breakfast cereals, pulses, bread, poultry, green vegetables, nuts and dried fruit, especially apricots.

Note that iron in animal foods is absorbed more easily by the body than iron from plant sources, but having vitamin C-rich fruit and vegetables with meals boosts iron absorption from plant sources. Tea, coffee and calcium supplements reduce iron absorption, so take these one hour before or after meals if you need to.

COMPLEMENTARY EXERCISE

Doing an additional form of exercise, often referred to as cross-training, is helpful in preventing or overcoming potential boredom from repeating the same activity. It also rests the muscles you are habitually using in your activities and gives others a workout. For example, if you usually walk or jog, try swimming, cycling or a weight-training class. Eventually you could be doing all three of the different types of exercise described on page 92 during a typical week. Such a varied regime will improve strength, flexibility and fitness, thereby increasing your 'core stability'. Having a stronger core (abdominal, lower back and pelvic muscles) stabilises the body and provides support for all movements.

METABOLISM AND YOU

The speed at which your body burns calories is your metabolic rate. This varies from person to person, even between individuals of the same size and age. Your resting (or base) metabolic rate (RMR) is the amount of calories your body consumes to keep it functioning at rest. For most people, RMR accounts for 70–85 per cent of the calories used each day.

Exercise can help raise your RMR, so you lose weight and fat more quickly. After aerobic exercise, for example, RMR is significantly elevated for up to $1\frac{1}{2}$ hours.

When working aerobically, your body is metabolising in the presence of oxygen. This is important because your body can burn fat as a fuel only if oxygen is present. If your goal is to lower your body-fat percentage or to lose weight, it makes sense to use body fat as a fuel. Everyone has a point in their aerobic zone (the range of heartbeat rate in which their body is working aerobically) where they are maximising the percentage of fat they are using for fuel.

As exercise intensity increases, such as progressing from a walk to a jog to a run to a sprint, the body's energy demands increase and the percentage of energy it obtains from burning fat decreases. This goes down until the anaerobic threshold (AT) is reached, where you stop burning body fat and all your energy demands are met by burning sugars (carbohydrates). This is called anaerobic glycolysis.

After you hit your AT you do not burn any more fat. For many people this happens very early on in an exercise session and explains why, despite working out hard and becoming very sweaty and breathless, some people cannot lose that final half stone of body fat. Paradoxically, they are working too hard to burn fat.

The way to change this is through long, slow-distance training at intensities lower than your anaerobic threshold. This increases your aerobic base and moves your AT higher, towards your maximum heart rate. This will enable you to work at higher intensities and still burn body fat.

To find your RMR and your anaerobic threshold, and to have a tailored exercise plan to target body-fat reduction by working within your aerobic heart rate zone, you need to consult a personal trainer or health club with access to the specialist equipment for taking the measurements.

Food for exercise

The rules are the same as for healthy eating. Fuel your activity with lots of starchy carbohydrates, at least five portions of fruit and vegetables a day, and moderate amounts of meat, fish and other protein foods, and dairy foods such as milk, yoghurt and cheese. Make sparing use of fats, oils and sugary foods, but if you regularly take vigorous exercise, you can probably get away with more sugary snacks than sedentary people. Bananas are great fuel for sport and exercise, but you could also enjoy low-fat sugary snacks, such as Jaffa cakes, jelly beans or cereal bars. Before a major endurance event, such as a marathon, competitors embark on 'carbohydrate loading' – trying to increase their stores of carbohydrates (and therefore energy) to the maximum.

You can do this yourself in a small way for something far less strenuous, such as a lunchtime trip to the gym. For example, if you have not eaten a meal since breakfast, have a light snack of one or two pieces of fruit about 45 minutes before your gym session.

After a workout, wait 40–60 minutes before eating, then have a carbohydrate-rich meal (pasta, rice, potatoes or bread) to replenish energy levels. Combine the carbs with a little protein, such as oily fish, lean red meat or poultry, nuts or another vegetarian alternative, and plenty of vegetables or a salad.

Remember to drink plenty of water before, during and after exercise – 1 litre/2 pints for every hour's training you do.

KEEPING TRACK

There is a variety of hardware available to help you monitor your body's performance when exercising. For example, heart-rate monitors can help you to work within specific heart-rate zones, ensuring that you burn fat and save yourself wasted effort. Some monitors are programmed to calculate your heart-rate zone and warn you to slow down or speed up, while others have built-in calorie counters and fitness tests to check your progress.

Different monitors are suited to different activities, so take care to choose one with your speciality in mind. Swimming, for example, will require one that's waterproof.

If you are a keen walker, a pedometer will let you know what distance you have covered.

Some monitors have memories, so you can track your progress over time, comparing how long it took to cover a specific distance on previous occasions. Others, such as chest-strap monitors, can be linked to gym equipment so that they transmit information to the screen of the treadmill or exercise bike.

Chapter 5
The diets

We all have plenty of reasons for why we put on weight: holidays, birthdays, Christmas, parties, 'addictions' to particular foods, 'friends' who lead us astray, sedentary jobs, vending machines at work, unhealthy canteen food, lack of money, genetic inheritance... Genuine or not, they're all excuses. The simple reason why we put on weight is because we eat more food than we need: we take in more calories than we burn. Losing and maintaining weight, as this book explains earlier, relies on finding an equilibrium between the calories we eat and the calories we use up by being a lot more active.

There are three ways in which the body burns up calories.

- Some 50–70 per cent of calories are used while the body is at rest. This might seem odd, but it takes energy to maintain normal body temperature and the work of the heart and intestinal muscles.
- About 10 per cent of calories are used by the body in the actual process of metabolising (burning) food.
- The remaining 20–40 per cent of calories are used up by physical activity, namely, everything else you do that takes more effort than lying down.

If you eat more than you need, your body stores the extra calories in fat cells. If you don't use up that extra energy through regular exercise and regulating the amount you eat, fat builds up and you become overweight. In addition, adults lose around 2 kg/5 lb of muscle every decade of their life, which leads to a 2–5 per cent decrease in metabolic rate because it's muscle, not fat, that burns calories. Given these facts, it becomes easier to see why many people gain around 6.5 kg/15 lb of fat every decade of their life – unless they exercise and eat moderately.

We all tend to put on weight with age, so we think it's normal to do so. It isn't. It's simply usual. We don't have to put on weight at all.

MOTIVATE YOURSELF

Losing pounds and looking better is a goal probably shared by most of the population. Achieving that goal is within reach of everyone, especially if you apply the principles of this book. The more challenging part is to bring about a permanent change in your eating habits and attitude. For this you need motivation, so here are a few tips for finding and maintaining it.

First, be resolved. You have to decide that you want to lose weight. If you are not committed, it will not happen. Once you have decided to lose weight, think about how you are going to do it. Consider the obstacles in your way and how you will overcome them.

Don't think about weight loss in isolation. Strengthen your resolve by also considering the health benefits of not being overweight: you will have a lower risk of disabling problems such as heart disease, diabetes and stroke.

Put nutrition before calories. This is the best pattern of eating for achieving weight loss. Think in terms of nutrient-dense foods rather than 'dieting' foods, and choose these options as you go for moderation rather than over-restraint in your eating.

Get everyone in the family on board. If you have a family, everyone will have to eat the same food, even if the quantities are different. You are more likely to stick to your diet if everyone is eating healthily. You will also be encouraging them to adopt healthier eating habits.

Find ways to enjoy physical activity. Recognise that being more active will help with weight loss and also reduce health risks. Having accepted that, work out ways to exercise regularly, or incorporate more activity into your day-to-day life. Frequent bursts of activity for as little as 10 minutes several times a day all add up to greater fitness and calorie burning.

Don't fixate on weight. Exercise replaces fat with muscle, so as you become fitter, you might not lose as much weight as you'd hoped. Remember, overall health and fitness are far more important than numbers on a scale. It's healthier to be overweight and fit than unfit and slim.

Set realistic goals. Don't try to lose more than 10 per cent of your body weight; 5 per cent is a reasonable goal. And avoid 'all or nothing' thinking. If you have failed at weight loss before, it doesn't matter. Don't be too strict or hard on yourself. Weight loss will take time, and weight lost slowly is weight lost more permanently.

Be careful about who you ask for support. Family and friends can be very good at undermining changes in diet and lifestyle because they challenge their own behaviour too.

Reward yourself for healthier eating. Avoid 'treats' such as chocolate and fast food, and opt instead for a magazine, book or CD – something you have wanted for ages – or bigger treats, such as saunas, facials, haircuts and new clothes. Or why not go on a few outings? A day's golf, a trip in a hot-air balloon, a scuba diving course... The possibilities are endless.

Stay off the scales. Don't weigh yourself more than once a week. Gradual weight loss of around 1 kg/2 lb a week is the best approach and is more likely to be permanent than faster weight loss. Remember that you may go through a period of no weight loss, so be honest with yourself and ask, 'Have I kept to my diet and been as physically active as I need to be?' If you have, don't be disheartened; in a couple of weeks you will continue your weight reduction.

NEW BODY, NEW THINKING

In order to win the new body that you want, you will have to acquire a new mindset. Given the widespread availability and persistent marketing of food, losing weight is not easy, especially if you are someone who craves food beyond normal appetite requirements. On many occasions you will need to be strong-minded in order to make the best choices for weight control and health.

If you are not committed to losing weight, it will not happen. Stay positive, stay strong and ask others for help if you need it. The effort will be worth it in the end.

Keep in mind an image of the new you, whether that person is slimmer, more toned or just healthier. Having goals for reducing weight and increasing activity will ease your way to making better food choices and changing your eating patterns. Don't feel discouraged if you slip off track now and again; praise yourself for all the times you have made healthier choices and the times you are going to do so in future.

If you are one of the many people with a 'dieting mentality' – a repetitive cycle of losing weight, regaining it and dieting again – congratulate yourself on leaving that behind you. You are now entering a new world of permanent weight loss, where you are going to commit to regular exercise and moderate food intake.

STAY ACTIVE

Building physical activity into the slimming and maintenance eating plans on the following pages is essential for health. A minimum of 30 minutes moderate activity a day, or on most days, is helpful to tip the energy balance towards weight loss and weight maintenance.

And be realistic: even if you are a bit overweight, it is better to be fit and overweight than unfit and too thin. If in any doubt, consult your doctor before starting any slimming plan.

RING THE CHANGES

- The plans and menus that follow are designed to include a wide variety of foods.

- Each day's eating contains at least five portions of fruit and vegetables, plus the protein and dairy foods needed for health, and a good amount of starchy carbohydrates.

- You can swap the menus around or repeat certain days, if you like. If you construct your own 28-day eating plan from the choices below, ring the changes as much as possible, and do not over-rely on any one type of food.

- If you find the daily allowance of calories too high for you to lose weight, you can reduce it, but by no more than 200 calories.

- Vegetarian options are included in all lunches and evening meals.

- Foods followed by an asterisk (*) have recipes in Chapter 6.

The 28-day slimming plan for women

1200 calories a day

Dairy/soya products: In addition to the milk you have with breakfast cereal, this plan also permits one of the following each day:

- 300 ml/10 fl oz skimmed milk
- 200 ml/7 fl oz semi-skimmed milk
- 200 ml/7 fl oz soya milk
- 125 ml/4 fl oz low-fat natural or fruit yoghurt
- 125 ml/4 fl oz low-fat fromage frais or similar soya dessert.

One option is to have a yoghurt on most days and a milky drink on others because few people will use all the milk allowance in hot drinks – so don't forget to use it all.

Spread should be used where indicated in the diet, such as for making sandwiches. However, if you prefer to swap spread for mayonnaise, for example, here are the options:

- 1 tsp standard margarine or butter
- 2 tsp low-fat spread
- 1 tsp vegetable oil (sunflower or olive)
- 1 tbsp low-fat mayonnaise.

Sandwiches should be made with two slices of thick-cut wholegrain bread.

Bread, potatoes, rice and pasta serving suggestions are given in each menu, but these are interchangeable, so swap them around as you prefer. However, as *Eat for Life* encourages a varied diet, try not to rely too much on any one type. Use the portion sizes listed below:

- 200 g/7 oz potatoes (uncooked weight)
- 50 g/2 oz fresh pasta (uncooked weight, equivalent to 90 g/3½ oz cooked weight)
- 40 g/1½ oz dry pasta (uncooked weight, equivalent to 135 g/4¾ oz cooked)
- 40 g/1½ oz rice (uncooked weight, equivalent to 125 g/4½ oz cooked weight, boiled)
- 2 slices thick-cut wholegrain bread

Vegetables to accompany main meals can be boiled, steamed, braised or prepared in any way that involves no added fat. Alternatively, serve them raw, if preferred. Standard portions are 80 g/3¼ oz, but if you feel especially hungry, you can fill up on a larger portion. For variety and specific portion information, see page 53.

Pudding is not served every day, but when it is, a choice may be made from the lists on page 111.

WEEK ONE

Monday

Breakfast: 1 glass unsweetened fruit juice, 3 tbsp Cheerios with 1 small banana

Mid-morning snack: 1 piece of fruit

Lunch: 15 cm/6 in piece French stick with green salad and 1 slice of lean ham or 1 small slice Emmental or Gruyère cheese

Mid-afternoon snack: 1 piece of fruit

Evening meal: 150 g/5 oz cod, haddock or other white fish steak or fillet topped with 1 tbsp pesto and grilled, steamed or fried in a non-stick pan without added fat, or Chickpea hotpot*; serve with 1 portion of potato and 2 portions of vegetables

Tuesday

Breakfast: 1 glass unsweetened fruit juice, 3 tbsp muesli with milk or yoghurt

Mid-morning snack: 1 piece of fruit

Lunch: 1 slice wholegrain toast topped with half a can of sardines in tomato sauce or about 75 g/3 oz mushroom pâté (or similar); serve with 125 g/4½ oz (half a tub) low-fat coleslaw

Mid-afternoon snack: 1 piece of fruit

Evening meal: Mexican tortilla* with crudité garnish

Pudding: Choose 1 from List A (see page 111)

Wednesday

Breakfast: 1 glass unsweetened fruit juice, 1 wholemeal hot-cross bun with spread

Mid-morning snack: 1 piece of fruit

Lunch: 1 large wholemeal pitta bread filled with 70 g/2 ¾ oz reduced-fat hummus, lettuce and carrot

Mid-afternoon snack: 1 piece of fruit

Evening meal: Spaghetti bolognese* or vegetarian option in recipe

Thursday

Breakfast: 1 glass unsweetened fruit juice, 1 Granary roll with 1 slice lean ham or 50 g/ 2 oz cottage cheese

Mid-morning snack: 1 piece of fruit

Lunch: Sandwich filled with 1 chopped hardboiled egg mixed with 2 tsp reduced-fat mayonnaise, plus chopped cress or watercress

Mid-afternoon snack: 1 piece of fruit

Evening meal: Salmon kedgeree* or vegetarian option in recipe

Friday

Breakfast: 1 glass unsweetened fruit juice, 5 tbsp Shreddies with milk

Mid-morning snack: 1 piece of fruit

Lunch: 1 corn on the cob with spread, Tabbouleh* and 70 g/2 ¾ oz reduced-fat mixed bean salad or canned mixed beans

Mid-afternoon snack: 1 piece of fruit

Evening meal: Chicken curry* or Butter bean and mushroom bake* with 1 portion of rice

Saturday

Breakfast: 1 glass unsweetened fruit juice, 3 Krisprolls or crispbreads with 2 tsp low-fat soft white cheese

Mid-morning snack: 1 piece of fruit

Lunch: Spinach mash* topped with 1 poached egg

Mid-afternoon snack: 1 piece of fruit

Evening meal: Fresh tuna salad* or vegetarian option

Pudding: Choose 1 from List B (see page 111)

Sunday

Breakfast: 1 glass unsweetened fruit juice, 1 slice raisin toast or fruit loaf with spread

Mid-morning snack: 1 piece of fruit

Lunch: Smoked haddock pie* or Spinach and cheese squares* with 2 portions of vegetables

Pudding: 1 yoghurt

Mid-afternoon snack: 1 piece of fruit

Evening meal: Tomato and mozzarella bruschetta*

WEEK TWO

Monday

Breakfast: 1 glass unsweetened fruit juice, 1 slice wholemeal bread with spread and 2 tsp marmalade or jam

Mid-morning snack: 1 piece of fruit

Lunch: 1 medium–large baked potato filled with 65 g/2½ oz tuna in oil with 3 tbsp sweetcorn kernels (no added sugar or salt variety), or half a 400 g /14 oz can of beans in chilli or spicy sauce

Mid-afternoon snack: 1 piece of fruit

Evening meal: Monkfish and bacon kebabs* with 1 portion of rice and 2 portions of vegetables, or Pepper and potato tortilla* with 2 portions of vegetables

Pudding: Choose 1 from List B (see page 111)

Tuesday

Breakfast: 1 glass unsweetened fruit juice, 1 medium slice white toast with 2 tsp peanut butter (no added salt or palm oil)

Lunch: 1 large baked potato filled with 40 g/ 1½ oz grated Cheddar or other hard cheese

Pudding: 1 piece of fruit

Evening meal: Pork kebab* with Yoghurt dip*, or vegetarian option in recipe, served with 1 portion of rice and 2 portions of vegetables

Evening snack: 1 piece of fruit

Wednesday

Breakfast: 1 glass unsweetened fruit juice, porridge made with milk and topped with 1 tsp syrup, black treacle or sugar

Mid-morning snack: 1 piece of fruit

Lunch: Carrot and nut salad* with wholemeal batch roll

Mid-afternoon snack: 1 piece of fruit

Evening meal: Simple prawn curry* or vegetarian option in recipe, served with 1 portion of rice

Pudding: Fruit brûlée*

Thursday

Breakfast: 1 glass unsweetened fruit juice, 1 low-fat muffin (cake type)

Mid-morning snack: 1 piece of fruit

Lunch: Macaroni cheese (1 portion reduced-fat, ready-made) served with 1 portion of vegetables

Pudding: Grilled peaches*

Evening meal: Mushroom risotto*

Evening snack: 1 piece of fruit

Friday

Breakfast: 1 x 250 ml/8 fl oz bottle of smoothie and a digestive or oat biscuit

Mid-morning snack: 1 piece of fruit

Lunch: 1 glass unsweetened fruit juice, sandwich filled with 1 chopped hardboiled egg mixed with 2 tsp reduced-fat mayonnaise, plus chopped cress or watercress

Evening meal: Salmon fishcake* or Spinach and cheese squares* served with 2 portions of vegetables

Pudding: 1 piece of fruit

Saturday

Breakfast: 1 glass unsweetened fruit juice, ½ grapefruit, 4 ready-to-eat prunes, 1 slice toast with spread

Mid-morning snack: 1 piece of fruit

Lunch: 1 medium slice (150 g/5 oz) pizza Margarita plus cereal bowl of mixed green salad with 1 tbsp French dressing

Mid-afternoon snack: 1 piece of fruit

Evening meal: Beef fillet or steak with 1 portion of potatoes and 2 portions of vegetables, or Stuffed pepper* with 1 portion of new potatoes (Tip: make double portions of the stuffed peppers and freeze for week four.)

Pudding: 1 yoghurt (from allowance) plus 1 Biscotti*

Sunday

Breakfast: 1 glass unsweetened fruit juice, 1 lean rasher grilled back bacon (not for vegetarians, who have a higher-calorie pudding later instead), 1 egg cooked without added fat, 1 grilled tomato, 1 medium slice wholemeal toast with scraping of spread

Mid-morning snack: 1 piece of fruit

Lunch: Tomato and mozzarella bruschetta*

Mid-afternoon snack: 1 piece of fruit

Evening meal: Griddled scallop salad* or vegetarian option in Fresh tuna salad* with 1 portion of potatoes

Pudding: Choose 1 from List A (see page 111); vegetarians can choose 1 from List B, as they had fewer calories at lunchtime

WEEK THREE

Monday

Breakfast: 1 glass unsweetened fruit juice, 2 tbsp muesli with 1 grated apple stirred in

Mid-morning snack: 1 piece of fruit

Lunch: Sandwich made with 2 slices lean roast beef, salad and 1 tsp horseradish mixed with the spread, or Tomato and courgette soup* with 2 Krisprolls

Mid-afternoon snack: 1 piece of fruit

Evening meal: 1 medium trout, grilled or steamed, served with 1 portion of rice and 2

portions of vegetables, or Vegetable curry* served with 1 portion of rice

Pudding: Choose 1 from List A (see page 111)

Tuesday

Breakfast: 1 glass unsweetened fruit juice, 4 tbsp granola with milk

Mid-morning snack: 1 piece of fruit

Lunch: 1 large baked potato filled with 200 g/ 7 oz (half a can) baked beans

Pudding: 1 low-fat fruit fool plus 1 Jaffa cake

Mid-afternoon snack: 1 piece of fruit

Evening meal: Burger* (no bap or salad) served with 1 portion of Ratatouille*; or purchase a vegetarian burger containing no more than 250 calories

Pudding: Choose 1 from List B (see page 111)

Wednesday

Breakfast: 1 glass unsweetened fruit juice, 1 wholemeal muffin (bread type) spread with 2 tsp lemon curd

Mid-morning snack: 1 piece of fruit

Lunch: Carrot and coriander soup* with 2 brown rice cakes or 1 large oatcake

Mid-afternoon snack: 1 piece of fruit

Evening meal: Salmon (or haddock) fishcake*, or Spinach and cheese squares*, served with 2 portions of vegetables

Thursday

Breakfast: 1 glass unsweetened fruit juice, 1 wholemeal roll and 1 Babybel cheese or 1 triangle of cheese spread

Mid-morning snack: 1 piece of fruit

Lunch: Sandwich made with 75 g/3 oz skinless roast chicken breast, green salad and 1 tsp reduced-fat mayonnaise, or Aubergine pâté* with 2 slices toast and green salad

Mid-afternoon snack: 1 piece of fruit

Evening meal: 1 white fish steak (150 g/5 oz) served with Tabbouleh* and 2 portions of vegetables, or Grilled summer vegetables* served with Tabbouleh* and 1 mini wholemeal roll

Pudding: Choose 1 from List A (see page 111)

Friday

Breakfast: 1 glass unsweetened fruit juice, 1 Weetabix with 2 tbsp raisins and milk

Mid-morning snack: 1 piece of fruit

Lunch: Sandwich made with 75 g/3 oz peeled cooked prawns in dressing made from 2 tsp low-fat mayonnaise and 1 tsp tomato ketchup, or sandwich spread with 1 tsp pesto and filled with grilled vegetables (peppers, courgettes, aubergine)

Mid-afternoon snack: 1 piece of fruit

Evening meal: Chicken and lime salad*, or vegetarian option in recipe, with 1 portion of new potatoes

Pudding: Choose 1 from List A (see page 111)

Saturday

Breakfast: 1 individual bottle Actimel, Yakult or similar probiotic drink with 1 medium wholegrain cereal bar, e.g. Jordan's Crunchy

Mid-morning snack: 1 piece of fruit
Lunch: 1 glass unsweetened fruit juice, 1 piece toast with spread and 1 poached egg

Mid-afternoon snack: 1 piece of fruit

Evening meal: Minestrone* served with 2 tbsp grated Parmesan, 1 green salad and 1 tbsp French dressing*

Sunday

Breakfast: 1 glass unsweetened fruit juice, 1 medium brioche spread with 2 tsp lemon curd

Mid-morning snack: 1 piece of fruit

Lunch: Chicken and walnut salad* or vegetarian option in recipe

Mid-afternoon snack: 1 piece of fruit

Evening meal: 1 boiled egg with 1 slice toast and spread

Pudding: 1 yoghurt (from daily allowance)

WEEK FOUR

Monday

Breakfast: 1 glass unsweetened fruit juice, 4 tbsp Raisin Wheats with milk

Mid-morning snack: 1 piece of fruit

Lunch: 1 bagel with 1 slice smoked salmon and 2 tsp low-fat soft white cheese, or with shavings of Parmesan and sliced tomato

Mid-afternoon snack: 1 piece of fruit

Evening meal: Spaghetti bolognese* or vegetarian option in recipe

Pudding: 1 yoghurt (from daily allowance)

Tuesday

Breakfast: 1 glass unsweetened fruit juice, 1 yoghurt with cereal corner

Mid-morning snack: 1 piece of fruit

Lunch: Lentil soup* with 1 wholemeal roll and spread

Mid-afternoon snack: 1 piece of fruit

Evening meal: 2 x 75g/3 oz chicken thighs (weight with bone) grilled and served with 1 portion of potato and 2 portions of vegetables, or Pasta salad*

Pudding: 1 yoghurt (from daily allowance) with 1 Biscotti*

Wednesday

Breakfast: 1 glass unsweetened fruit juice, 3 tbsp Cheerios with milk and 1 small banana

Mid-morning snack: 1 piece of fruit

Lunch: 200 g/7 oz (half a can) baked beans on 1 slice toast

Pudding: 1 digestive biscuit served with 1 yoghurt (from allowance)

Mid-afternoon snack: 1 piece of fruit

Evening meal: Smoked haddock pie* served with 2 portions of vegetables, or Courgette risotto* served with 1 large green salad and French dressing*

Thursday

Breakfast: 1 glass unsweetened fruit juice, 5 tbsp Shreddies with milk

Mid-morning snack: 1 piece of fruit

Lunch: 1 large baked potato with 100g/4 oz (half a tub) vegetable pasta sauce

Mid-afternoon snack: 1 piece of fruit

Evening meal: Carrot and coriander soup* with 1 wholemeal roll

Pudding: 1 Jaffa cake served with yoghurt (from allowance)

Friday

Breakfast: ½ grapefruit, 4 prunes, 1 slice wholemeal toast with spread

Mid-morning snack: 1 piece of fruit

Lunch: 1 glass unsweetened fruit juice, cheese and pickle sandwich made with 40 g/1½ oz grated cheese, 1 sliced tomato and 1 tsp pickle or chutney

Mid-afternoon snack: 1 piece of fruit

Evening meal: Fresh tuna salad* or Mexican tortilla*, served with 1 portion of new potatoes

Pudding: Choose 1 from List A (see right)

Saturday

Breakfast: 1 glass unsweetened fruit juice, porridge made from 40 g/1½ oz porridge oats and milk from allowance, plus 1 tsp syrup or black treacle

Mid-morning snack: 1 piece of fruit

Lunch: 15 cm/6 in piece French stick with 1 slice lean ham or 1 small slice Emmental or Gruyère cheese, and green salad,

Pudding: 1 low-fat yoghurt

Mid-afternoon snack: 1 piece of fruit

Evening meal: Griddled scallop salad* with 1 portion new potatoes, or Bean salad* served with 1 wholemeal roll

Pudding: Choose 1 from List A (see above)

LIST A PUDDINGS
- Fruit kebab* plus 2 Biscotti*
- Grilled peaches*
- Brioche and red berries*
- Strawberry coeur à la crème*
- Fresh figs and raspberry coulis*
- Strawberry and amaretti crunch*
- 2 scoops mango sorbet*, no Biscotti

LIST B PUDDINGS
- Hot fruit salad*
- Pears in red wine*
- Vanilla yoghurt sundae*
- 3 scoops mango sorbet* plus 1 Biscotti*
- Barbecued fruit*
- Rock cake*

Sunday

Breakfast: 1 glass unsweetened fruit juice, 1 wholemeal muffin (bread type) with 2 tsp lemon curd or jam

Mid-morning snack: 1 piece of fruit

Lunch: 100 g/4 oz grilled steak, with 1 portion of potatoes and 2 portions of vegetables, or Stuffed pepper* with green salad and 1 tsp French dressing*

Pudding: Choose 1 from List A (see above)

Mid-afternoon snack: 1 piece of fruit

Evening meal: Lentil soup* plus 2 rice cakes

The 28-day slimming plan for men and 28-day maintenance plan for women

1700 calories a day

This plan is for men who want to lose weight and women who want to maintain weight loss. It works on a simple 'top-up' principle, adding the extra calorie requirement to the previous 1200-calorie slimming plan. If you find the daily allowance of 1700 calories too high for you to lose weight, you can reduce it, but by no more than 200 calories.

Women who have lost weight with the 1200-calorie diet and wish to maintain that weight loss can do so if they follow this 1700-calorie diet.

Dairy/soya products: The daily allowance is the same as for the 1200-calorie diet, which was:
- 300 ml/10 fl oz skimmed milk
- 200 ml/7 fl oz semi-skimmed milk

- 200 ml/7 fl oz soya milk
- 125 ml/4 fl oz low-fat natural or fruit yoghurt
- 125 ml/4 fl oz low-fat fromage frais or similar soya dessert.

Bread, rice, pasta and potatoes: To make up the 1700-calorie plan, you are allowed either 2 of the carbohydrate portions listed below, or 1 of these and a pudding from the list right.
- 200 g/7 oz potatoes (uncooked weight)
- 50 g/2 oz fresh pasta (uncooked weight, equivalent to 90 g/3½ oz cooked weight)
- 40 g/1½ oz dry pasta (uncooked weight, equivalent to 135 g/4¾ oz cooked)

- 40 g/1½ oz rice (uncooked weight, equivalent to 125 g/4½ oz cooked weight, boiled)
- 2 slices thick-cut wholegrain bread
- 1 wholemeal hot-cross bun
- 1 Rock cake*

Additional fruit and vegetables: Add 1 extra portion each day of fruit or vegetables (see portion guides, pages 53 and 58).

Puddings: If you have a sweet tooth, you can have 1 of the following puddings in place of 1 of the additional starchy food servings above.
- Fruit kebab* and 1 Biscotti*
- Grilled peaches*
- Brioche and red berries*
- Strawberry coeur à la crème*
- 2 scoops mango sorbet* and 1 Biscotti*
- Fresh figs with raspberry coulis*

Snacks: On the 1700-calorie eating plan, you are allowed 2 snacks a day from the list opposite.

SNACKS FOR 1,700 CALORIE DIETS

- 1 digestive biscuit
- 1 fig roll
- 1 slice malt loaf, unspread
- 25 g/1 oz reduced-fat Edam cheese
- 1 mini hot-cross bun, no spread
- 250 ml/8 fl oz carrot juice
- 3 breadsticks (grissini)
- 1 milk chocolate Hobnob
- 1 Hovis digestive
- 1 standard glass (200 ml/7 fl oz) lager, bitter, cider
- 1 standard glass (125 ml/4 fl oz) dry white wine (11% alcohol)
- 1 pub measure (25 ml/1 fl oz) spirit, plus low-calorie mixer
- 6 whole almonds
- 1 choc ice
- Flavoured cottage cheese spread on 1 Ryvita
- 2 crackers or biscuits for cheese
- 100 g/4 oz low-fat custard
- 2 fresh dates with stones or 1 Medjool date
- 2 dried figs
- 3 fresh figs
- 1 small pot (100 g/4 oz) fromage frais
- 1 fruit lolly
- 2 Jaffa cakes
- 1 regular skinny latte or cappuccino
- 1 pot (60–70 g/2½–2¾ oz) low-fat or diet chocolate mousse
- 1 large oatcake
- 2–3 slices pastrami
- 2 prawn toast canapés
- 2 thick rice cakes
- 1 chicken satay stick
- 1 chipolata or 2 cocktail sausages
- 1 mini Scotch/savoury egg
- 1 tbsp sunflower or pumpkin seeds
- 5 slices wafer-thin turkey or ham
- 3 prawn dim sum wontons
- 2 scoops mango sorbet*
- fruit kebab*
- 2 Biscotti*
- 1 low-fat fruit yoghurt

The seven-day maintenance plan

2000 calories a day

Mainly for men, but also suitable for extremely active women who do at least one hour of vigorous activity per day.

Daily allowances: The following allowances are not included in the menus below, so add them during the day when it suits your appetite.
- 2 portions of fruit
- 300 ml/10 fl oz skimmed milk, or 200 ml/ 7 fl oz semi-skimmed milk, or 200 ml/7 fl oz soya milk
- 125 ml/4 fl oz low-fat natural yoghurt or fat-free fruit yoghurt

Spread should be used where indicated in the diet, such as for making sandwiches. However, if you prefer to swap spread for mayonnaise, for example, here are the options: 1 tsp standard margarine or butter or 2 tsp low-fat spread or 1 tsp vegetable oil (sunflower or olive) or 1 tbsp low-fat mayonnaise.

Sandwiches should be made with two slices of thick-cut wholegrain bread.

Bread, potatoes, rice and pasta serving suggestions are given in each menu, but these carbohydrates are interchangeable, so swap them around as you prefer. However, as *Eat for Life* encourages a varied diet, try not to rely too much on any one type. Use the portion sizes listed below:
- 200 g/7 oz potatoes (uncooked weight)
- 50 g/2 oz fresh pasta (uncooked weight, equivalent to 90 g/3½ oz cooked weight)
- 40 g/1½ oz dry pasta (uncooked weight, equivalent to 135 g/4¾ oz cooked)
- 40 g/1½ oz rice (uncooked weight, equivalent to 125 g/4½ oz cooked weight, boiled)
- 2 slices thick-cut wholegrain bread

Each day of the following eating plans will provide at least 5 portions of fruit and vegetables, a good balance of protein and dairy foods, plus starchy carbohydrates such as bread, potatoes, pasta and rice.

Monday

Breakfast: 100 ml/3½ fl oz orange juice, 1 thick slice wholemeal toast with scraping of spread and 2 tsp marmalade or jam, 45 g/1¾ oz breakfast cereal, e.g. Shreddies, with 125 ml/4 fl oz semi-skimmed milk (from allowance)

Lunch: Sandwich containing 75 g/3 oz skinless roast chicken or 1 chopped hardboiled egg, plus tomato, lettuce and 2 tsp reduced-fat mayonnaise

Main meal: Fresh tuna salad* or Mexican tortilla* served with 1 portion of new potatoes

Pudding: Choose from list B (see page 116)

Snacks: Choose 2 from list on page 116

Tuesday

Breakfast: ½ grapefruit and 4 prunes, 100 ml/3½ fl oz orange juice, 1 thick slice wholemeal toast with scraping of spread and 2 tsp marmalade or jam

Mid-morning snack: 1 yoghurt with cereal corner

Lunch: 225 g/8 oz baked potato filled with 150 g/5 oz baked beans plus 1 slice ham (not for vegetarians, who have a higher-calorie pudding instead), green salad and tomato

Main meal: Chicken or vegetarian chop suey*

Pudding: Choose 1 from List A (see page 116), or List B for vegetarians to make up the calories they missed in the ham

Snack: Choose 1 from list on page 116

Wednesday

Breakfast: 100 ml/3½ fl oz orange juice, 1 thick slice wholemeal toast with scraping of spread and 2 tsp marmalade or jam, 50 g/2 oz muesli with milk from allowance

Lunch: Sandwich containing 75 g/3 oz tuna in water, 50 g/2 oz low-fat soft cheese and 1/3 diced pepper, or 50 g/2 oz reduced-fat hummus and 1 large grated carrot

Main meal: Burger* (purchase vegetarian version if preferred) in bap with green salad and 1 tbsp French dressing*

Pudding: Choose 1 from List B (see page 116)

Snack: Choose 1 from list on page 116

Thursday

Breakfast: 3 tbsp fruit compote or fruit salad with 125 g/4½ oz low-fat vanilla yoghurt, 2 small slices raisin bread or similar fruit loaf with scraping of spread

Mid-morning snack: 1 Frusli or small cereal bar

Lunch: 1 large floury wholemeal bap filled with 50 g/2 oz reduced-fat mozzarella cheese, 1 sliced tomato, lettuce and shredded basil leaves, served with 50 g/2 oz olives

Main meal: Meatballs with red pepper sauce* and 1 portion of pasta; vegetarians can replace the meatballs with felafels (rissoles made of mashed chickpeas)

Pudding: Choose 1 from List B (see page 116)

Snacks: Choose 2 from list on page 116

Friday

Breakfast: 100 ml/3½ fl oz orange juice, 1 wholemeal muffin (bread type), hot-cross bun or scone, or fruited teacake, plus spread and 2 tsp jam or honey

Mid-morning snack: 1 mini (60 g/2¼ oz) low-fat fromage frais and 1 large banana

Lunch: Lentil soup* garnished with 1 tbsp low-fat natural yoghurt, plus 10 cm/4 in piece of French stick

Main meal: Liver and bacon* with 1 portion of potato and 2 portions of vegetables, or Mushroom risotto* with 1 large mixed salad and 1 tbsp French dressing*

Pudding: Choose 1 from List B (see page 116)

Snack: Choose 1 from list on page 116

Saturday

Breakfast: 1 x 250 ml/8 fl oz bottle of smoothie, 1 reduced-fat muffin (cake type) or 1 reduced-fat croissant with 2 tsp honey

Lunch: Salad leaves with ½ small avocado, 50 g/2 oz peeled prawns in Marie Rose dressing (1 tsp reduced-fat mayonnaise mixed with 1 tsp tomato ketchup), plus 1 portion new potatoes; for a vegetarian option, omit the prawns and dress the potatoes with 50 g/2 oz low-fat soft white cheese flavoured with garlic and chopped herbs of choice

Main meal: Sweet and sour pork* (vegetarian option available) with 1 portion of rice

Pudding: Choose 1 from List B (see below)

Snack: Choose 1 from list below

Sunday

Breakfast: 100 ml/3½ fl oz orange juice, 1 thick slice wholemeal toast, 1 lean grilled back rasher (not for vegetarians, who have a higher-calorie pudding later instead), 1 grilled tomato, 1 fried egg (cooked in nonstick pan without added fat)

Mid-morning snack: 1 toasted teacake with scraping of spread

Main meal: 1 x 150 g/5 oz grilled lamb leg steak served with Spinach mash*, or Kedgeree variation* and Ratatouille*

Pudding: Choose 1 from List B (see below)

Supper: Minestrone* with 10 cm/4 in piece French stick

Snack: Choose 1 from list below

LIST A PUDDINGS
- Fruit kebab* and 2 Biscotti*
- Grilled peaches*
- Brioche and red berries*
- Strawberry coeur à la crème*
- Fresh figs and raspberry coulis*
- Strawberry and amaretti crunch*

LIST B PUDDINGS
- Hot fruit salad*
- Pears in red wine*
- Vanilla yoghurt sundae*
- Mango sorbet*
- Barbecued fruit*
- Rock cake*

SNACKS
- 1 Weetabix biscuit with 125 ml/4 fl oz semi-skimmed milk
- 50 g/2 oz wholegrain breakfast cereal with skimmed milk
- 1 small serving (100 g/4 oz) porridge
- 1 matchbox-sized piece (40g/1½ oz) cheese
- 300 ml/10 fl oz semi-skimmed milk
- 1 x 250 ml/8 fl oz bottle of smoothie
- 1 wholemeal hot-cross bun (bread type)
- 1 wholemeal scone
- 1 wholemeal muffin
- 1 rock cake*
- 1 cereal bar
- 3 Jaffa cakes
- 2 oat biscuits
- 2 digestive biscuits
- 2 fig rolls
- 2 small pieces malt loaf
- 1 small packet crisps
- 1 bowl carrot and coriander soup* with oatcake
- 2 mini muffins

Chapter 6
Recipes

Many of the recipes in this chapter are used within the diet plans in Chapter 5, but they are also intended for everyday use. Their ingredients reflect the basic principles of healthy eating, which are highlighted overeleaf so that you can adjust the recipes you use at the moment and the way you prepare your food to help with weight loss or maintaining your ideal weight.

Tips for healthy cooking

- As a general rule, steam, bake, boil, poach, grill, dry roast or microwave food when it requires cooking.
- Keep frying to a minimum, and use the smallest amount possible of added fat.
- Cut off all visible fat from meat.
- Avoid, or use only rarely, fatty meat products, such as sausages, pâtés and pies.
- Choose unsaturated vegetable oils, such as sunflower and soya.
- Avoid hard and saturated fats such as lard, ghee, dripping, block margarines, coconut milk and creamed coconut.
- Skim fat from stocks and soups before serving. (If made the day before needed and allowed to become cold, the fat will rise to the top and set, making it easier to remove.)
- Replace processed foods with fresh foods, particularly fruit and vegetables, whenever you can.
- Choose wholemeal and wholegrain ingredients for your cooking whenever possible. There is nearly three times more fibre in wholemeal flour than white flour, five times more fibre in brown rice than white, and more than double the fibre in wholemeal pasta than plain egg pasta.
- Swap full-fat milk, cream and cheese for lower-fat products, such as skimmed milk and yoghurt.
- Make generous use of spices and herbs instead of adding salt.
- Be sparing with stock cubes, soy sauce and other sauces because they are high in salt. Try salt-free or low-sodium versions.
- Limit your use of salted foods, such as bacon, anchovies and olives.

Minimise vitamin and mineral loss

To get the maximum goodness from fruit and vegetables it is best to eat them raw: simply wash and eat. When you need to cook them, do the preparation just before they go in the pot. Scrub rather than peel them, where appropriate, to preserve the nutrients and fibre in the skin, and don't chop them too small as that exposes more surfaces to the air and results in nutrient loss. To minimise this loss, dress cut surfaces immediately with lemon juice, or a minimal amount of unsaturated vegetable oil if you plan to roast or grill them.

Steaming vegetables is the best way to preserve their nutrients, but if you boil them, do so for the shortest time possible in the minimum amount of water. Minerals from the vegetables leach into the cooking water, so save it and use for soups and sauces.

Sweet enough

You know by now that sugar is an empty food, providing calories but no nutrients, so try to cut down on it in your cooking. Most recipes can be adjusted to reduce the sugar content. In fact you can cut out up to 20 per cent in baked goods.

There is generally no need to add sugar when cooking fruits (except, perhaps, rhubarb and gooseberries, which are very tart). If extra flavour is required, try adding vanilla or spices such as cinnamon, cardamom, allspice, cloves and nutmeg. Purées of dried fruit, such as peaches, pears, apricots and prunes, make a good substitute for sugar in recipes as the drying process intensifies their sweet flavour.

How to make your own healthy eating plans

Making your own eating plans doesn't mean that you have to write out menus for the week ahead, but there is no harm in doing so if you want to. It is enough to think about each day as a unit in which you try to balance your food intake. You may already do this subconsciously, but most of us need to make an effort to get into this habit.

Thinking ahead applies largely to the two main meals of the day, and boils down to balancing one meal against another. If, for example, one contains fish or meat, then the other need not do so. If one is quite large, make the other smaller. If possible, try to eat most of your calories early in the day rather than going without and then having a large meal in the evening when you have less time to digest it.

BREAKFAST

Eating breakfast gives you a head start in terms of vitamin and mineral intake, and research has shown that non-breakfast-eaters are unlikely to make up that difference during the day. Another effect of going without breakfast is a tendency to eat larger meals and have a higher intake of fatty and sugary foods throughout the rest of the day.

Regular breakfast-eaters have been shown to perform better because breakfast raises energy levels and improves concentration. They score higher in memory and concentration tests, and – perhaps best of all – tend to be more cheerful.

What should you have for breakfast? Well, cereals, especially fortified ones, are rich in B vitamins, including folic acid, and minerals such as iron (good for energy). Folic acid reduces the risk of heart disease by lowering raised levels of homocysteine, and protects pregnant women against birth defects such as spina bifida.

The milk poured over the cereal is also a good source of the B vitamin riboflavin, vitamin B_{12} for energy, and calcium for strong bones. If you prefer soya milk, choose a fortified version.

Breakfast is a great opportunity to increase fibre intake and prevent constipation, so choose wholegrain cereals, porridge, prunes and other dried fruit. Fibre also reduces the risk of heart attack by lowering blood cholesterol, and the fermentation of fibre by-products in the gut improves immune function.

Can't get through to lunch without a snack? Eat a piece of fruit or a low-fat yoghurt.

LUNCH AND DINNER

Before you eat lunch think about what you will have for dinner. That doesn't mean deciding exactly what's going to be on the menu; it just means thinking ahead to balance your diet. For example, if you are going to eat a main meal later in the day, have a light lunch.

Both meals should be based on the following healthy eating principles: plenty of fruit and vegetables, lots of starchy, high-fibre foods, such as bread, rice, pasta and potatoes, moderate amounts of lean protein (meat, fish or vegetarian), and low amounts of fat. Eating a wide variety of foods makes for a more interesting and enjoyable diet. It also makes for a healthier diet because you receive a wider range of vitamins and minerals. While you know by now that it's wise to reduce the amount of fat you consume, it is not a good idea to cut out fat entirely. Some fat (preferably unsaturated from oily fish, nuts and seeds) is essential for health (see the portion guidelines below).

Portion guide

If you find it helpful to think in terms of portions, try to make your everyday meals (not special meals for high days and holidays) from the following daily amounts, but remember that the portions required of some food groups, e.g. carbohydrates and fats, depend on each individual's energy requirements.

Carbohydrates: 6–11 portions per day. 1 portion = 3 tbsp breakfast cereal or 1 roll or 1 slice of bread or 2 tbsp cooked potato, rice, pasta or noodles.

Fruit and vegetables: at least 5 portions per day. 1 portion = 80 g/3¼ oz or 3 tbsp cooked or canned produce or 1 cereal bowl of salad or 1 piece of fresh fruit or 100 ml/3½ fl oz fruit juice. For detailed guides, see pages 53 and 58.

Milk, cheese and yoghurt: 2–3 portions per day. 1 portion = 200 ml/7 fl oz milk or 40 g/1½ oz hard cheese or 120 g/4½ oz yoghurt or fromage frais.

Meat, fish and alternatives: 2–3 portions per day. 1 portion = 50–75 g/2–3 oz meat, poultry or oily fish or 100–150 g/4–5 oz white fish or 3 fish fingers or 1–2 eggs or 3 tbsp cooked beans, lentils or other pulses, or 2 tbsp nuts or peanut butter.

Fats: up to 5 portions per day, including fatty foods (cream, crisps, pastry, sausages and other fatty meat products). 1 portion = 1 tsp butter, margarine, oil or mayonnaise or 2 tsp low-fat spread.

RECIPES

- Note that all spoonfuls are level.
- Use either metric or imperial measures, not a mixture of both.
- The calorie and nutrient information following each recipe is per serving. It does not include the suggestions for carbohydrate and vegetable accompaniments.
- The symbol √ indicates vegetarian recipes.

LUNCHES

Tabbouleh √

Serves 2

50 g/2 oz bulgur (cracked wheat)
1 small or ½ large cucumber, deseeded and
  diced
1/3 green pepper, deseeded and finely diced
2 spring onions, diced
2 tbsp freshly chopped mint
juice of ½ lemon
freshly ground black pepper

1. Cook the bulgur in twice its volume of
   boiling water for 10 minutes, or leave to
   stand in the same amount of just-boiled
   water for 15 minutes until the grain has
   swelled and softened. Drain, if necessary.
2. Transfer the bulgur to a serving bowl and
   stir in the remaining ingredients.

Per serving
Calories: 103
Protein: 3.2 g
Carbohydrates: 22 g, of which sugars = 2.8 g
Fat: 0.6 g, of which saturates = trace
Sodium: trace
Fibre: 0.7 g

Tomato and Mozzarella Bruschetta √

Serves 2

½ ciabatta loaf or 2 ciabatta rolls
1 garlic clove, peeled and halved
1 tbsp extra virgin olive oil
2 ripe plum tomatoes, sliced
1 tbsp shredded basil leaves
120 g/4 ½ oz pack reduced-fat mozzarella
  cheese, drained and sliced
6 black olives, to garnish
freshly ground black pepper, to serve

1. Preheat the grill to medium. Halve the bread
   or roll lengthways. Toast the bread lightly,
   then rub the garlic clove over the cut side
   and drizzle with the olive oil.

2. Arrange the tomatoes and basil on the
   bread, top with the mozzarella and grill
   again until the cheese has melted.

3. Garnish with the olives and serve, offering
   black pepper separately.

Per serving
Calories: 341
Protein: 17.9 g
Carbohydrates: 33.8 g, of which sugars =
   4.5 g
Fat: 15.1 g, of which saturates = 5.4 g
Sodium: 0.75 g
Fibre: 2.5 g

Carrot and Nut Salad √

Serves 4

450 g/1 lb carrots, peeled
75 g/3 oz natural roasted nuts, e.g. peanuts,
    cashews or pistachios
2 large handfuls parsley, chopped
2 tbsp orange juice
2 tbsp French dressing (see page 142)
freshly ground black pepper

1. Combine all the ingredients and serve.

Per serving
Calories: 185
Protein: 5.4 g
Carbohydrates: 8.4 g, of which sugars = 7.4 g
Fat: 14.7g, of which saturates = 2.5 g
Sodium: 0.2 g
Fibre: 4.8 g

Spinach and Cheese Squares √

Serves 4

2 large eggs
100 g/4 oz wholemeal flour
275 g/10 oz frozen chopped spinach, thawed
    and drained well
450 g/1 lb cottage cheese
175 g/6 oz reduced-fat Cheddar cheese
freshly ground black pepper

1. Preheat the oven to 180°C/350°F/Gas
   mark 4.

2. Beat the eggs and flour together in a large
   bowl. Add the spinach, cottage cheese,
   Cheddar and black pepper.

3. Spoon the mixture into a well-greased,
   large ovenproof dish and bake for about 45
   minutes.

4. Leave to cool for at least 5 minutes, until
   slightly firmed, before cutting into squares and
   serving.

Per serving
Calories: 329
Protein: 36.2 g
Carbohydrates: 22.2 g, of which sugars = 4.2 g
Fat: 11.5 g, of which saturates = 5.5 g
Sodium: 0.8 g
Fibre: 2.2 g

Aubergine Pâté √

Serves

2 medium aubergines
2 garlic cloves, crushed
1 tbsp vegetable oil
2 tbsp orange juice
1 tsp paprika
pinch chilli powder

1. Preheat the oven to 180°C/350°F/Gas
   mark 4.

2. Prick the aubergines with a fork and place
   on a baking tray. Bake for 45 minutes or
   until tender.

3. When the aubergines are cooked, remove
   the skin as soon as cool enough to handle.

4. Purée the flesh in a food processor with the
   rest of the ingredients. Chill before serving.

Per serving

Calories: 66

Protein: 1.4 g

Carbohydrates: 7.1 g, of which sugars = 6. 0g

Fat: 3.9 g, of which saturates = 0.5 g

Sodium: trace

Fibre: 4.4 g

Bacon and Pasta Soup
Serves 2

1 celery stick, diced
1 onion, diced
1 garlic clove, crushed
3 rashers lean back bacon, diced
400 g/14 oz can tomatoes
120 ml/4 fl oz vegetable stock or water
75 g/3 oz pasta shells
2 carrots, grated
2 tbsp freshly chopped parsley

1. Place the celery, onion, garlic and bacon in a pan over a low heat, cover and sweat for about 3 minutes. Stir occasionally to prevent sticking.

2. Add the tomatoes and stock and cook for 10 minutes, breaking up the tomatoes.

3. Add the pasta and cook until *al dente*.

4. Remove the mixture from the heat, and stir in the carrot and parsley before serving.

Per serving

Calories: 262

Protein: 14.8 g

Carbohydrates: 45.3 g, of which sugars = 14.8 g

Fat: 3.6 g, of which saturates = 1 g

Sodium: 0.84 g

Fibre: 6.6 g

Lentil Soup √
Serves 4

75 g /3 oz split red lentils
50 g/2 oz dried apricots
300 g/11 oz sweet potato, peeled and chopped
1 litre/1¾ pints vegetable stock
2 tsp lemon juice

1. Wash the lentils and put in a pan with the apricots, sweet potato and stock. Bring to boiling point, then reduce the heat and simmer for 20 minutes.

2. Transfer to a blender or food processor and liquidise to the desired consistency.

3. Add the lemon juice and reheat gently before serving.

Per serving

Calories: 156

Protein: 7.1 g

Carbohydrates: 32.4 g, of which sugars = 10.2 g

Fat: 0.7 g, of which saturates = 0.1 g

Sodium: 0.37 g

Fibre: 3.7 g

Carrot and Coriander Soup √

Serves 4

60 g/2½ oz split red lentils
2 tbsp olive oil
1 onion, chopped
1 large potato, scrubbed and cubed
375 g/13 oz carrots, scrubbed and cubed
900 ml/1½ pints vegetable stock
1 packet fresh coriander, chopped
grating of fresh nutmeg (optional)

1. Rinse the lentils and put in a saucepan. Cover with boiling water and leave for 10 minutes while you prepare the vegetables.

2. Heat the oil in a large heavy-bottomed pan, and sauté the onion for 5 minutes.

3. Add the potato, carrots, lentils in their soaking water and stock. Bring to the boil, lower the heat and simmer for 20 minutes until everything is very soft.

4. Transfer to a blender or food processor and liquidise to the desired consistency.

5. Return the soup to the pan, add the coriander and reheat very gently.

6. Check the seasoning, adding a little grated nutmeg if you like.

Per serving
Calories: 183
Protein: 6.5 g
Carbohydrates: 26.8 g, of which sugars = 9.8 g
Fat: 6.3 g, of which saturates = 0.8 g
Sodium: 0.33 g
Fibre: 3.9 g

Tomato and Courgette Soup √

Serves 4

2 tsp sunflower oil
1 large onion, peeled and chopped
2 cloves garlic, crushed
400 g/14 oz can tomatoes
450 g/1 lb courgettes
450 ml/15 fl oz water
2 tbsp tomato purée
1 tsp sugar
large handful basil, chopped
1 tbsp wine vinegar
freshly ground black pepper

1. Heat the oil in a large saucepan and cook the onion and garlic until soft, stirring frequently, about 5–8 minutes.

2. Add all the other ingredients, and simmer for 20–25 minutes until the vegetables are tender.

3. Purée the soup in a blender and serve.

Per serving
Calories: 88
Protein: 4.1 g
Carbohydrates: 12.5 g, of which sugars = 7.0 g
Fat: 3.0 g, of which saturates = 0.3 g
Sodium: trace
Fibre: 1.8 g

Minestrone √

Serves 2

1 tbsp olive oil
1 large onion, diced
2 garlic cloves, crushed
2 carrots, diced
2 celery sticks, chopped
73 g/3 oz French beans, sliced
1 courgette, sliced
225 g/8 oz ripe tomatoes, chopped, or
    200 g/ 7 oz canned tomatoes in natural
    juice
600 ml/1 pint vegetable stock
1 tsp fresh thyme leaves
200 g/7 oz cooked cannellini beans, drained
    and rinsed
50 g/2 oz macaroni or other small pasta
    shapes for soup
2 tbsp chopped fresh parsley
freshly ground black pepper
2 tbsp grated Parmesan, to serve

1. Heat the oil in a large saucepan, add the onion and garlic and fry until they begin to soften.

2. Add the remaining vegetables up to and including the tomatoes. Stir well.

3. Pour in the stock, bring to the boil, then cover and simmer for about 30 minutes until all the vegetables are tender.

4. About 15 minutes before the end of cooking, add the cannellini beans, the pasta, parsley and seasoning.

5. Sprinkle each serving with 1 tbsp Parmesan.

EAT SOUP TO LOSE WEIGHT

Soup is liquid, so its volume fills you up for fewer calories (provided it is not full of double cream and butter). Hot soup also has to be eaten slowly, which allows time for the appetite mechanism to tell you that the stomach is full. This prevents you overeating, which is what happens when food is eaten too quickly.

Home-made soup is a marvellous standby meal, so make it in large quantities and freeze in individual portions for future use.

Per serving
Calories: 378 (411 if served with Parmesan)
Protein: 17.4 g
Carbohydrates: 61.6 g, of which sugars = 23.3 g
Fat: 8.6 g, of which saturates = 1 g
Sodium: 0.50 g
Fibre: 13.8 g

MAIN MEALS

Salmon Fishcakes
Serves 2

200 g/7 oz salmon fillet
250 g/9 oz cold mashed potato
1 tbsp chopped fresh dill
1 tbsp reduced-calorie mayonnaise
freshly ground black pepper
4 tbsp skimmed milk (optional)
40 g/1½ oz fine breadcrumbs
1 tbsp oil, for frying

1. Put the salmon in a saucepan with enough water almost to cover. Bring to simmering point and poach for 5 minutes. Drain and cool, then flake the flesh, discarding the skin and bones.

2. Mash the fish with the potato, dill, mayonnaise and seasoning, then form the mixture into four small cakes.

3. Dip the cakes in milk (if you like) before rolling them in the breadcrumbs, and fry lightly in hot oil for 4 minutes on each side.

Variation: Other types of fish may be used in place of salmon. Try smoked haddock (uncoloured), and increase the quantity to 350 g/12 oz as it contains fewer calories than salmon.

Per serving
Calories: 414
Protein: 25 g
Carbohydrates: 37.7 g, of which sugars = 1.8 g
Fat: 19.1 g, of which saturates = 3.2 g
Sodium: 0.35 g
Fibre: 2 g

Simple Prawn Curry
Serves 2

1 tbsp vegetable oil
2 onions, diced
2 garlic cloves, crushed
1 green chilli, deseeded and diced
400 g/14 oz large ripe tomatoes, chopped
½ tsp ground cumin
½ tsp coriander
150 g/5 oz cooked peeled prawns

1. Heat the oil and fry the onion, garlic and chilli for 5 minutes, until transparent but not browned.

2. Add the tomatoes and spices, then cover and cook over a moderate heat for a further 15 minutes, until the tomatoes have softened and amalgamated.

3. Stir in the prawns and cook for a further 2–3 minutes, until they have heated through.

Variation: Vegetarians can replace the prawns with 25 g/1 oz cashew nuts.

Per serving
Calories: 206
Protein: 20.4 g
Carbohydrates: 15.7 g, of which sugars = 11.9 g
Fat: 7.3 g, of which saturates = 0.9 g
Sodium: 1.22 g
Fibre: 3.6 g

Monkfish and Bacon Kebabs

Serves 2

100 g/4 oz spinach leaves
4 rashers lean back bacon, trimmed of fat
225 g/8 oz monkfish or other firm white fish,
    cut into 8 chunks
8 cherry tomatoes

1. Blanch the spinach leaves by plunging them into boiling water for 2 minutes. Drain and press out the excess moisture.

2. Flatten and stretch the bacon by using a round-bladed knife. Cut each rasher in half across the middle.

3. Put a layer of spinach leaves on each piece of bacon, top with a chunk of fish and wrap the bacon round to form a little parcel.

4. Thread the bacon-wrapped fish on to skewers, alternating the 'parcels' with tomatoes.

5. Preheat the grill until very hot, then grill the kebabs for about 8 minutes, turning frequently until thoroughly cooked.

Per serving
Calories: 153
Protein: 27.5 g
Carbohydrates: 2.1 g, of which sugars = 2.1 g
Fat: 4 g, of which saturates = 1.3 g
Sodium: 0.84 g
Fibre: 1.5 g

Griddled Scallop Salad

Serves 2

1 tsp sesame oil
2 tbsp lime juice
pinch ground chilli
2 tbsp fresh chopped coriander
50 g/2 oz rocket or lamb's lettuce
200 g/7 oz scallops, with or without roes

1. Mix the oil, lime juice, chilli and coriander and whisk thoroughly.

2. Pour one third of the dressing over the salad leaves, toss well, then set aside.

3. Preheat the grill to a medium-high heat.

4. Put the remaining dressing in a shallow ovenproof dish and add the scallops, turning to coat.

5. Place the dish under the heat and grill for 5–6 minutes, turning occasionally to prevent burning.

6. When cooked, place on top of the dressed salad leaves and serve at once.

Per serving
Calories: 114
Protein: 20.1 g
Carbohydrates: 1.1 g, of which sugars = 0.4 g
Fat: 3.3 g, of which saturates = 0.6 g
Sodium: 0.23 g
Fibre: 0.4 g

Salmon Kedgeree

Serves 2

1 tbsp vegetable oil
½ tsp ground cumin
5 green cardamom pods, bruised
100 g/4 oz basmati rice, washed
½ tsp turmeric powder
450 ml/15 fl oz water or fish stock
225 g/8 oz salmon tail, skinned and cut into
    chunks
25 g/1 oz flaked almonds, toasted
1 tbsp chopped fresh coriander or flat-leaf
    parsley
2 free-range eggs, hardboiled and sliced, to
    garnish

1. Heat the oil, add the cumin and cardamom
   pods and fry for a couple of minutes.

2. Stir in the rice and cook until golden.

3. Add the turmeric and the water or fish
   stock and stir well. Cover the pan and cook
   on a very low heat for 15 minutes.

4. Add the salmon and continue cooking until
   the liquid has been absorbed and the rice is
   cooked – about another 10 minutes.

5. Remove from the heat and stir in the
   almonds and coriander.

6. Garnish with slices of egg and a few extra
   coriander leaves. Serve hot or cold.

Variation: Vegetarians can replace the salmon
with 50 g/2 oz dried apricots, and replace the
fish stock with vegetable stock. Add the
apricots when the salmon would have been
added. Stir in an additional 25 g/1 oz flaked
almonds and sultanas at the end of the recipe.

Per serving
Calories: 559
Protein: 33.3 g
Carbohydrates: 42.5 g, of which sugars = 0.6 g
Fat: 29.6 g, of which saturates = 4.4 g
Sodium: 0.13 g
Fibre: 0.9 g

Fresh Tuna Salad

Serves 2

6 waxy salad potatoes, scraped and halved
4 tbsp French dressing (see page142)
1 garlic clove, crushed
75 g/3 oz French beans, boiled
2 plum tomatoes, quartered
1 crispy lettuce heart, leaves separated
4 anchovy fillets, drained
2 free-range eggs, hardboiled and quartered
120 g/4½ oz tuna steak, grilled
8 black olives

1. Boil the potatoes until just cooked. Drain
   and transfer to a large bowl.

2. Mix the salad dressing with the garlic, then
   pour half of it over the warm potatoes.

3. Add the beans and tomatoes and toss the
   mixture well.

4. Place the lettuce leaves in the base of 2
   serving dishes.

5. Flake the tuna over the leaves, then top
   with the anchovy fillets, egg quarters and
   olives.

Variations: Mackerel or salmon may be used instead of tuna, if preferred.

Vegetarians can replace the anchovy fillets and tuna with 100 g/4 oz marinated and grilled artichoke hearts and 28 g/1 oz walnut pieces.

Per serving
Calories: 344 (without dressing)
Protein: 27.4 g
Carbohydrates: 33.8 g, of which sugars = 6.8 g
Fat: 11.9 g, of which saturates = 2.9 g
Sodium: 0.63 g
Fibre: 4.1 g

Smoked Haddock Pie
Serves 2

225g/8 oz potatoes, peeled and cut into
    chunks
50 ml/ 2 fl oz skimmed milk
1 tbsp horseradish sauce
2 tbsp fresh dill, chopped
300 g/11 oz smoked haddock, skinned
50 g/2 oz frozen peas
150 ml/5 fl oz reduced-fat crème fraîche

1. Preheat the oven to 200°C/400°F/Gas mark 6.

2. Boil the potatoes until tender, then drain and return them to the pan.

3. Add the milk and horseradish sauce, then mash well. Stir in the dill.

4. Cut the fish into chunks and put in an ovenproof dish with the peas and the crème fraîche.

5. Spoon the mash over the fish mixture and level the top, then bake in the oven for 30 minutes until the surface is nicely brown.

Per serving
Calories: 368
Protein: 36.1 g
Carbohydrates: 27.8 g, of which sugars = 6.6 g
Fat: 13.3 g, of which saturates = 7.4 g
Sodium: 1.31 g
Fibre: 3 g

Chicken Chop Suey
Serves 2

100 g/4 oz plain egg noodles
2 tbsp vegetable oil
300 g/11 oz chicken, cut into thin strips
1 tsp cornflour
4 tbsp soy sauce
¼ tsp ground ginger
1 tbsp wine vinegar
juice of 1 orange
150 ml/5 fl oz water
200 g/7 oz pak choi leaves, shredded
100 g/4 oz beansprouts
4 spring onions, sliced
100 g/4 oz canned bamboo shoots or water
    chestnuts, thinly sliced

1. Put the noodles on to boil or steam. Drain when cooked, then cover and keep warm.

2. Heat the oil in a wok or large pan and fry the chicken for 5 minutes.

3. Mix together the cornflour, soy sauce, ginger, vinegar, orange juice and water to make a smooth paste.

4. Add the vegetables and cornflour mixture to the pan and continue cooking, stirring occasionally, for another 10 minutes.

5. Halfway through the cooking time, mix in the noodles, heat through and serve at once.

Variation: Vegetarians can replace the chicken with Quorn chunks or tofu.

Per serving

Calories: 528

Protein: 47.2 g

Carbohydrates: 49 g, of which sugars = 8.1 g

Fat: 17.4 g, of which saturates = 2.2 g

Sodium: 2.53 g

Fibre: 1.5 g

CHICKEN CURRY

Serves 2

1 tbsp vegetable oil

1 onion, sliced

½ red pepper, deseeded and sliced

1 garlic clove, crushed

1 tsp ground cumin

1 tsp ground coriander

½ tsp chilli powder (optional)

½ tsp ground turmeric

225 g/8 oz chicken breast, skinned, boned and cut into strips

½ tsp cornflour

2 tbsp water

120 ml/4 fl oz natural low-fat yoghurt

150 ml/5 fl oz chicken stock

1 tsp garam masala

1. Heat the oil, then fry the onion, pepper and garlic for about 5 minutes until transparent but not browned.

2. Add the spices and the chicken, and continue cooking for another 5 minutes, stirring to prevent the mixture sticking to the pan.

3. Mix the cornflour with the water to make a smooth paste, then combine it with the yoghurt.

4. Stir the stock into the chicken mixture and simmer gently for 5 minutes.

5. Stir in the yoghurt and garam masala and heat through for a couple of minutes before serving.

Per serving

Calories: 266

Protein: 32.8 g

Carbohydrates: 15 g, of which sugars = 9 g

Fat: 8.6 g, of which saturates = 1.5 g

Sodium: 0.22 g

Fibre: 1.4 g

Chicken and Walnut Salad

Serves 2

1 small iceberg lettuce heart, leaves
   separated
50 g/2 oz baby spinach leaves
2 tbsp French dressing made with walnut oil
   (see page 142)
1 large chicken breast, skinned, boned,
   cooked and sliced
75 g/3 oz walnut halves
75 g/3 oz chopped dates
50 g/2 oz raisins

1. Toss the lettuce and spinach leaves in the
   dressing.

2. Arrange the leaves on a serving dish, then
   scatter the chicken, nuts and raisins on top.

Variation: Vegetarians can replace the
chicken with half a large avocado, sliced.

Per serving
Calories: 596
Protein: 29.4 g
Carbohydrates: 45.4 g, of which sugars = 44.7 g
Fat: 34.2 g, of which saturates = 4.1 g
Sodium: 0.12 g
Fibre: 4 g

Chicken and Lime Salad

Serves 2

2 chicken breasts, skinned and boned
1 tsp olive oil
freshly ground black pepper
1 iceberg lettuce heart, leaves separated
½ cucumber
2 tbsp chopped fresh coriander
2 tbsp chopped fresh mint
1 tsp sesame oil
2 tbsp lime juice
4 spring onions, chopped

1. Preheat the grill to a medium heat.

2. Brush the chicken breasts with the olive oil,
   season with pepper and grill on both sides
   until cooked. Slice or shred the meat, and
   place in a large bowl with the lettuce.

3. Deseed the cucumber and chop finely. Mix
   with the herbs, sesame oil, lime juice and
   spring onions. Add to the lettuce and
   chicken and toss well.

Variation: Vegetarians can replace the
chicken with 25 g/1 oz lightly toasted pine
nuts and 1 skinned and sliced red pepper (see
Tip, page 134).

Per serving
Calories: 210
Protein: 35.4 g
Carbohydrates: 3.9 g, of which sugars = 3.1 g
Fat: 6 g, of which saturates = 1.1 g
Sodium: 0.09 g
Fibre: 1.2 g

Spaghetti Bolognese

Serves 2

1 onion, finely diced
1 celery stick, finely chopped
225 g/8 oz extra lean minced beef
1 carrot, finely chopped
400 g/14 oz can chopped tomatoes in
    natural juice
1 tsp tomato purée
1 bay leaf
1 tbsp chopped fresh parsley
150 ml/5 fl oz meat or vegetable stock
50 g/2 oz spaghetti (dry weight) per person

1. Put the onion, celery and beef in a non-stick pan and cook over a moderate heat for 5 minutes to brown the meat.

2. Add the carrot, tomatoes and tomato purée, the bay leaf, parsley and stock and stir well. Simmer for 20 minutes over a low heat, stirring occasionally to prevent sticking.

3. During the last 10 minutes of cooking time, boil the spaghetti until *al dente*, then drain and transfer to a serving dish.

4. Remove the bay leaf from the sauce and spoon over the pasta.

Variation: Vegetarians can make the sauce with Quorn or soya vegetable protein.

Per serving
Calories: 439
Protein: 34.6 g
Carbohydrates: 50.7 g, of which sugars = 12.9 g
Fat: 12.3 g, of which saturates = 4.9 g
Sodium: 0.39 g
Fibre: 5.8 g

Low-fat Burgers

Serves 2

225 g/8 oz lean minced beef (less than
    10 per cent fat)
1 onion, diced
1 large carrot, grated
1 tsp Dijon mustard
freshly ground black pepper
2 baps
1 tomato, sliced
lettuce

1. Put the meat, onion, carrot and mustard in a bowl and mix well. For a finer mixture, blend these ingredients in a food processor.

2. Form the mixture into 2 burgers.

3. Preheat the grill until very hot, then grill the burgers for about 8 minutes on each side.

4. Place each burger inside a bap with some lettuce and slices of tomato.

Per serving
Calories: 385 for burger in bap (240 for burger alone)
Protein: 31 g (25.8 g)
Carbohydrates: 36 g (9.3 g), of which sugars = 10.9 g (7.4 g)
Fat: 14.1 g (11.4 g), of which saturates = 5.4 g (4.7 g)
Sodium: 0.47 g (0.19 g)
Fibre: 3.6 g (2.1 g)

Meatballs with Red Pepper Sauce

Serves 2

200 g/7 oz extra lean minced lamb
1 large onion, chopped
2 garlic cloves, crushed
1 tbsp fresh coriander, chopped
1 tbsp tomato purée
freshly ground black pepper
50 g/2 oz pasta per person, to serve

Red pepper sauce

2 tsp olive oil
2 small onions, chopped
2 red peppers, deseeded and chopped
leaves from 2 sprigs thyme
200 ml/7 fl oz vegetable stock

1. Place all the meatball ingredients in a food processor, add seasoning, then purée to a smooth mixture.

2. Lightly flour your hands and form the mixture into balls. Set aside, or in the fridge, until needed.

3. To make the sauce, heat the oil in a pan and gently cook the onions for about 5 minutes, until softened but not browned.

4. Add the peppers and cook for a further 4 minutes.

5. Stir in the thyme, vegetable stock and some black pepper and cook for 20 minutes.

6. Purée the sauce in a blender until smooth.

7. Boil your chosen pasta.

8. While the pasta is cooking, preheat the grill until it is very hot. Grill the meatballs until golden brown, turning them often to cook evenly.

9. When the pasta is *al dente*, drain and transfer to a serving dish. Top with the meatballs and pour over the red pepper sauce.

Per serving
Calories: 193 for meatballs (87 for red pepper sauce)
Protein: 22 g (2 g)
Carbohydrates: 9.4 g (8 g), of which sugars = 6.2 g (8 g)
Fat: 7.8 g (5.5 g), of which saturates = 3.6 g (0.7 g)
Sodium: 0.29 g (trace)
Fibre: 1.7g (2.4 g)

Pork Kebab

Serves 2

225 g/8 oz minced lean pork
1 onion, chopped
1 garlic clove, peeled and crushed
1 chilli, deseeded and chopped
2 tsp tomato purée
1 tbsp fresh coriander leaves
1 tbsp fresh parsley
12 cherry tomatoes
1 red pepper, peeled and deseeded (see Tip on page 134)

1. Put all the ingredients except the tomatoes and red pepper in a food processor or mixing bowl and combine well.

2. Form the paste into balls, then arrange alternately on four skewers with the tomatoes and chunks of pepper.

3. Heat the grill or barbecue until very hot, then cook the kebabs for 10–15 minutes, turning frequently.

Variation: Vegetarians can use 200 g/7 oz Quorn in place of the pork, marinating it in the sweet and sour sauce (minus the cornflour) from the next recipe for about 1 hour.

Tip

To peel a pepper, impale it on a large fork and chargrill over a flame, or cut in half and place under a hot grill (skin side up), or microwave in a covered dish for 4–5 minutes. The skin will peel off easily, leaving just the softened flesh.

Per serving

Calories: 200
Protein: 27 g
Carbohydrates: 12 g, of which sugars = 10.3 g
Fat: 5.2 g, of which saturates = 1.5 g
Sodium: 0.10 g
Fibre: 2.9 g

Sweet and Sour Pork

Serves 2
1 tbsp vegetable oil
300 g/11 oz lean pork fillet, cut into thin strips
1 garlic clove, crushed or finely sliced
Chinese leaves or curly kale leaves, shredded
100 g/4 oz mange-tout
2 carrots, cut into sticks
1 red pepper, deseeded and sliced

Sweet and sour sauce

3 tbsp soy sauce
2 tsp cornflour
150 ml/5 fl oz orange juice
1 tsp tomato purée
1 tsp demerara sugar
1 tbsp wine vinegar

1. Heat the oil in a large wok and stir-fry the pork strips for 2 minutes.

2. Add the rest of the ingredients and continue cooking until the vegetables are almost cooked to the crispness you prefer.

3. Combine the soy sauce with the cornflour to make a paste, then stir in the remaining sauce ingredients.

4. Pour the sauce over the vegetables and heat through. The sauce will thicken as it cooks.

Variation: Vegetarians can replace the pork with Quorn chunks or tofu.

Tip

The sweet and sour sauce can also be used as a marinade if you omit the cornflour.

Per serving

Calories: 375
Protein: 37.9 g
Carbohydrates: 30.7 g, of which sugars = 24.4 g
Fat: 11.9 g, of which saturates = 2.5 g
Sodium: 1.64 g
Fibre: 5.4 g

Liver and Bacon

Serves 2

1 tbsp olive oil
2 onions, sliced
2 carrots, sliced
2 rashers lean back bacon, fat removed
1 tsp redcurrant or cranberry jelly
1 tsp tomato purée
225 g/8 oz lamb's liver

1. Heat the oil and fry the onions and carrots for 5 minutes, until softened but not brown.

2. Add the bacon and cook for a further 5 minutes.

3. Stir in the redcurrant jelly and tomato purée and add 4 tbsp water. Stir well and heat to simmering point.

4. Add the liver, then cover the pan. Simmer for up to 10 minutes, until the liver is cooked.

Per serving
Calories: 309
Protein: 28.7 g
Carbohydrates: 17 g, of which sugars = 14.2 g
Fat: 14.4 g, of which saturates = 3.3 g
Sodium: 0.49 g
Fibre: 3.6 g

Chickpea Hotpot √

Serves 4

2 tsp olive oil
1 large onion, peeled and chopped
2 garlic cloves, crushed
1 large aubergine, diced
2 red peppers, deseeded and sliced
1 tbsp paprika
400 g/14 oz can chickpeas, drained
100 g/4 oz mushrooms, sliced
400 g/14 oz can chopped tomatoes
1 sprig thyme
3 tbsp tomato purée
2 tbsp water
1 tsp ground cinnamon
freshly ground black pepper

1. Heat the oil in a large casserole. Add the onion and cook over a low heat for 10 minutes or until translucent.

2. Add the garlic and cook for a further 2 minutes, but do not allow to brown.

3. Add the aubergine and peppers, cover with a lid and cook for a further 5 minutes.

4. Stir in all the remaining ingredients, and simmer for 45 minutes, or until cooked.

Per serving
Calories: 184
Protein: 11.4 g
Carbohydrates: 29 g, of which sugars = 11.9 g
Fat: 3.5 g, of which saturates = 0.4 g
Sodium: trace
Fibre: 10.5 g

Mushroom Risotto √
Serves 2

25 g/1 oz dried mushrooms, e.g. porcini,
   morels or ceps
1 tbsp olive oil
50 g/2 oz fresh chestnut mushrooms, sliced
1 onion, chopped
1 celery stick, chopped
120 g/4 $\frac{1}{2}$ oz risotto rice, e.g. arborio or
   carnaroli
pinch saffron strands or $\frac{1}{2}$ tsp ground turmeric
600 ml/1 pint vegetable stock
freshly ground black pepper
grated Parmesan, to serve

1. Soak the dried mushrooms in water for
   about 15 minutes or according to the
   packet instructions. Strain, reserving the
   liquid, and chop any large mushrooms.

2. Heat the oil, add the fresh mushrooms,
   onion and celery, and fry gently for
   5 minutes.

3. Stir in the rice and saffron or turmeric, and
   cook, stirring, for a further 5 minutes, or
   until the rice is opaque.

4. Gradually add the drained mushrooms plus
   the stock and mushroom liquid, stirring
   between each addition. Simmer for about
   15 minutes until much of the liquid is
   absorbed. (Risotto is supposed to be
   creamy and moist, so do not let the mixture
   dry out.)

5. Serve, sprinkling each serving with 2 tbsp
   of Parmesan.

Variation: Broad beans or other vegetables
may be used in place of the mushrooms.

Per serving
Calories: 324 (357 if served with Parmesan)
Protein: 8.5 g
Carbohydrates: 61.4 g, of which sugars = 9.3 g
Fat: 6.6 g, of which saturates = 1 g
Sodium: 0.35 g
Fibre: 2.2 g

Butter Bean and Mushroom Bake √
Serves 4

225 g/8 oz dried butter beans, cooked, or
   600 g/1 lb 5 oz canned butter beans,
   drained
1 tbsp lemon juice
freshly ground black pepper
1 tsp sunflower oil
225 g/8 oz mushrooms, sliced
25 g/1 oz vegetable margarine
25 g/1 oz wholemeal flour
300 ml/10 fl oz water
25 g/1 oz Cheddar cheese, grated
25 g/1 oz fresh wholemeal breadcrumbs

1. Soak the dried butter beans for at least
   4 hours. Drain and cook in a pan of
   unsalted boiling water for 50–60 minutes or
   until tender. Drain.

2. Preheat the oven to 180°C/350°F/Gas
   mark 4.

3. Put the beans in a large, greased ovenproof
   dish. Add the lemon juice and black
   pepper.

4. Heat the oil in a pan and sauté the mushrooms until they soften, then add to the dish.

5. Heat the margarine in a nonstick pan, stir in the flour and cook for 2 minutes over a low heat, stirring continuously. Slowly add the water, and heat until thickened to a pouring consistency.

6. Pour the sauce over the beans and mushrooms.

7. Combine the cheese and breadcrumbs and sprinkle over the dish. Cook for 25 minutes.

Per serving
Calories: 275
Protein: 14.9 g
Carbohydrates: 34.6 g, of which sugars = 2.6 g
Fat: 9.6 g, of which saturates = 2.8 g
Sodium: 0.2 g
Fibre: 10.1 g

Mexican Tortilla √
Serves 2

75 g/3 oz cooked borlotti or brown beans, rinsed and drained
2 large ripe tomatoes, chopped
2 flour tortillas
1 small red onion, diced
2 tbsp chopped fresh coriander or parsley
1 small red chilli, finely diced
40 g/1½ oz Cheddar cheese, grated
chopped cucumber, radish and watercress, to garnish
2 tbsp reduced-fat crème fraîche, to serve

1. Mash the beans and tomatoes to a thick paste.

2. Spread half the paste in a thickish strip down the centre of each open tortilla. Top with the onion, coriander, chilli and cheese, then fold the tortilla over the filling, tucking in the sides, to make a sausage shape.

3. Wrap each filled tortilla in kitchen paper to hold it together, then cook on full power in a microwave oven for 1 minute 30 seconds. Alternatively, wrap in foil and cook in an oven preheated to 180°C/350°F/Gas mark 4 for 10–15 minutes.

4. Serve the tortillas topped with the garnishes and a blob of crème fraîche.

Per serving
Calories: 333
Protein: 13.9 g
Carbohydrates: 41.4 g, of which sugars = 7.2 g
Fat: 13.6 g, of which saturates = 6.3 g
Sodium: 0.93 g
Fibre: 4.5 g

Pepper and Potato Tortilla √
Serves 1

2 eggs
2 tsp water
freshly ground black pepper
2 tsp vegetable oil or margarine
75 g/3 oz cooked potato, sliced
50 g/2 oz red pepper, deseeded and diced

1. Preheat the grill to a moderate heat.
2. Break the eggs into a bowl, add the water and black pepper, and whisk lightly.

3. Heat the fat in a small nonstick frying pan, then pour in the egg mixture. Tilt the pan as the mixture cooks so that the runny parts slide under the set parts.

4. When the omelette is browned underneath but still moist on top, scatter the potato and pepper over it, then place under the grill to cook until lightly golden.

Per serving
Calories: 320
Protein: 17 g
Carbohydrates: 15.9 g, of which sugars = 1.4 g
Fat: 21.4 g, of which saturates = 5.7 g
Sodium: 0.3 g
Fibre: 1.2 g

Stuffed Peppers √
Serves 4

225 g/8 oz long-grain brown rice or bulgur
4 large green peppers, cut in half and
    deseeded
2 tsp olive or vegetable oil
2 onions, peeled and diced
2 garlic cloves, crushed
3 tbsp tomato purée
4 tbsp red wine, optional
75 g/3 oz cashew nuts, roughly chopped
400 g/14 oz canned tomatoes
2 tbsp fresh parsley, chopped
1 tbsp fresh thyme, chopped
freshly ground black pepper

1. Cook the rice in your usual way. If using bulgur, cover with water and boil for 10 minutes, or leave to soak for 15 minutes, according to the packet instructions. Drain if necessary.

2. Bring a large pan of water to the boil, put in the peppers and simmer for 5 minutes. Drain and place the peppers, cut side up, in a greased ovenproof dish.

3. Heat the oil in a large nonstick pan and sauté the onions until softened but not browned.

4. Add the garlic and cook for a further 2 minutes.

5. Add all the remaining ingredients except the rice, and simmer for 20 minutes.

6. Preheat the oven to 180°C/350°F/Gas mark 4.

7. Add the rice or bulgur to the onion mixture and stir thoroughly. Stuff the peppers with the mixture, placing any extra around them. Bake for 25 minutes.

Per serving
Calories: 288
Protein: 8.9 g
Carbohydrates: 36.2g, of which sugars = 10.8 g
Fat: 12.5 g, of which saturates = 0.4 g
Sodium: trace
Fibre: 4.2 g

Vegetable Curry √

Serves 4

1 tbsp sunflower or soya oil
1 large onion, peeled and chopped
2 celery sticks
2 garlic cloves, crushed
4 cloves
4 whole green cardamoms
1 tsp ground cumin
½ tsp ground coriander
½ tsp ground turmeric
1 tsp paprika or pinch chilli powder
1 parsnip, scrubbed and chopped
450 g/1 lb potatoes, scrubbed and chopped
1 courgette, sliced
½ small cauliflower, broken into florets
100 g/4 oz frozen peas
400 g/14 oz canned tomatoes, chopped
4 tbsp water

1. Heat the oil in a large flameproof casserole and cook the onion and celery over a low heat for 10 minutes, until softened.

2. Add the garlic and spices and cook for a further 2 minutes over a low heat.

3. Mix in all the vegetables and the water, cover and cook gently over a low heat for 35 minutes until tender.

Per serving
Calories: 205
Protein: 6.9 g
Carbohydrates: 36.6g, of which sugars = 7.1g
Fat: 4.7g, of which saturates = 0.5 g
Sodium: trace
Fibre: 7.8g

Grilled Summer Vegetables √

Serves 4

2 small aubergines
3 courgettes
1 yellow pepper, deseeded
1 red pepper, deseeded
1 tbsp olive oil
1 tbsp wine vinegar
1 garlic clove, crushed
1 tsp fresh oregano, chopped
freshly ground black pepper

1. Cut the aubergine into 5 mm/¼ in slices. Cut the courgettes diagonally into 1 cm/½ in slices. Cut each pepper into eight pieces.

2. Mix the oil, vinegar, garlic, oregano and black pepper in a large bowl. Add the vegetables and leave to marinate for at least 1 hour.

3. Heat the grill to a moderate heat.

4. Arrange the vegetables on a grill pan and grill until just tender, turning once or twice, and basting with the marinade from time to time.

Per serving
Calories: 95
Protein: 3.5 g
Carbohydrates: 11.7 g, of which sugars = 7.0 g
Fat: 4.5 g, of which saturates = 0.6 g
Sodium: trace
Fibre: 5.2 g

Pasta Salad √

Serves 4

1 lettuce, washed and dried
450 g/1 lb cooked wholemeal pasta
225 g/8 oz canned sweetcorn (no added salt
    or sugar), drained
1 apple, cored and diced
2 tomatoes, chopped
1 courgette, sliced
1 packet basil leaves, torn
4 tbsp French dressing (see page 142)
freshly ground black pepper

1. Line a salad bowl with the lettuce.

2. Toss all the remaining ingredients together,
    then place in the lined bowl and serve.

Per serving

Calories: 225
Protein: 6.4 g
Carbohydrates: 34.4 g, of which sugars = 12.0 g
Fat: 2.7 g, of which saturates = 0.9 g
Sodium: trace
Fibre: 5.2 g

Courgette Risotto √

Serves 4

2 tsp vegetable oil
1 small onion, peeled and sliced
1 garlic clove, crushed
350 g/12 oz courgettes, sliced
350 g/12 oz risotto rice
1.5 litres/2½ pints vegetable stock
1 packet fresh parsley, chopped
1 tbsp grated Parmesan cheese

1. Heat the oil in a large saucepan and cook
    the onion and garlic until soft.

2. Add the courgettes and cook for 7 minutes,
    stirring occasionally.

3. Add the rice, stirring until coated with oil,
    and cook for 1 minute until slightly opaque.

4. Stir in the stock, a ladleful at a time, waiting
    for each one to be absorbed before adding
    the next. Keep stirring between additions to
    prevent the rice sticking to the pan.

5. When all the stock has been added and the
    rice is tender (about 20 minutes), stir in the
    parsley and Parmesan.

Variation: Use 275 g/10 oz leeks, washed
and sliced, in place of the courgettes.

Per serving

Calories: 278
Protein: 7.4 g
Carbohydrates: 29.5 g, of which sugars =11.0 g
Fat: 14.7 g, of which saturates = 1.6 g
Sodium: 0.4 g
Fibre: 4.4 g

Bean Salad √

Serves 4

350 g/12 oz French beans, trimmed
400 g/14 oz cooked red kidney beans
225 g/8 oz cooked chickpeas

Dressing

1 tbsp Greek-style yoghurt
pinch sugar
freshly ground black pepper
1 tbsp chopped fresh mint
1 tsp French mustard
1 tbsp olive oil
2 tsp wine vinegar

1. Steam the French beans until just tender –
   about 5 minutes.

2. Drain and place in a large salad bowl with
   the kidney beans and chickpeas.

3. Mix the dressing ingredients together and
   pour over the beans. Toss to cover, then
   allow to stand for 1 hour before serving to
   let the flavours infuse.

Per serving

Calories: 157
Protein: 9.9 g
Carbohydrates: 21.8 g, of which sugars =
   3.2 g
Fat: 4.1 g, of which saturates = 0.6 g
Sodium: trace
Fibre: 11.3 g

Spinach Mash √

Serves 2

225 g/8 oz potatoes, peeled and chopped
90 g/3¼ oz fresh spinach leaves
2 tsp extra virgin olive oil
2 tsp lemon juice
freshly ground black pepper

1. Boil the potatoes until tender.

2. While the potatoes are cooking, wash the
   spinach, put in a covered pan and cook for
   3–4 minutes, until wilted. Drain well.

3. Drain the potatoes, reserving 50 ml/2 fl oz
   of the cooking water.

4. Mash the potatoes with the reserved water,
   olive oil and lemon juice.

5. Season to taste, and stir the spinach lightly
   into the mash to give a thickly marbled
   effect.

Per serving

Calories: 132
Protein: 3.6 g
Carbohydrates: 20.2 g, of which sugars =
   1.4 g
Fat: 4.6 g, of which saturates = 0.7 g
Sodium: 0.07 g
Fibre: 2.4 g

Ratatouille √

Serves 4

2 tbsp olive oil
1 aubergine, about 350 g/12 oz, cubed
2 courgettes, about 350 g/12 oz, sliced
2 red onions, sliced
1 green pepper, deseeded and cut into strips
1 red pepper, deseeded and cut into strips
225 g/8 oz tomatoes, chopped
2 tsp herbes de Provence (a mixture of
    rosemary, bay, basil and savory)
freshly ground black pepper

1. Heat the oil and fry the aubergine,
   courgettes, onions and peppers in a large
   pan until softened, stirring occasionally.

2. Add the tomatoes and herbs, then cover
   and reduce the heat. Cook gently for 20
   more minutes.

3. Check the seasoning before serving.

Per serving
Calories: 127
Protein: 4.1 g
Carbohydrates: 13.2 g, of which sugars = 11 g
Fat: 6.8 g, of which saturates = 0.9 g
Sodium: 0.01 g
Fibre: 5 g

DRESSINGS AND DIPS

French Dressing √
Serves 2

2 tbsp extra virgin olive oil or nut oil, e.g.
    walnut or hazelnut
2 tbsp wine, cider or sherry vinegar or lemon
    juice
½ tsp Dijon mustard
freshly ground black pepper

1. Combine all the ingredients and mix well.

Variation: Add 2 tbsp chopped fresh
tarragon, parsley, basil, mint, oregano or
coriander to the basic dressing.

Per serving
Calories: 103
Protein: 0.15 g
Carbohydrates: 0.5 g of which sugars = 0.2 g
Fat: 11.1 g, of which saturates = 1.5 g
Sodium: 0.04 g
Fibre: none

Soy Sauce Dressing √
Serves 2

1 tsp chopped or grated fresh ginger root
1 garlic clove, crushed
1 tsp sesame oil
2 tsp sunflower oil or other bland vegetable oil
1 tbsp soy sauce
1 tsp dry sherry

1. Combine all the ingredients and mix well.

Per serving

Calories: 70

Protein: 0.5 g

Carbohydrates: 1.35g, of which sugars = 0.75 g

Fat: 6 g, of which saturates = 0.53 g

Sodium: 0.53 g

Fibre: 0.1 g

Spicy Salad Dressing √

Serves 2

2 tbsp extra virgin olive oil or nut oil, e.g.
    walnut or hazelnut
2 tbsp white wine vinegar
½ tsp Dijon mustard
1 garlic clove, crushed
pinch chilli powder

1. Combine all the ingredients and mix well.

Per serving

Calories: 105

Protein: 0.4 g

Carbohydrates: 0.8 g, of which sugars = 0.25 g

Fat: 11.2 g, of which saturates = 1.5 g

Sodium: 0.1 g

Yoghurt Dip √

150 ml/5 oz low-fat natural yoghurt
1 tbsp chopped fresh mint
1 tbsp chopped fresh parsley
generous pinch ground cumin or 2 tsp
    toasted cumin seeds (see Tip)

1. Combine the yoghurt, herbs and cumin and
   mix well.

Tip

To toast the cumin seeds put them in a pan
without added fat and gently heat until lightly
brown.

Per recipe

Calories: 114

Protein: 9.5 g

Carbohydrates: 16.7 g, of which sugars = 16.7 g

Fat: 1.5 g, of which saturates = 0.8 g

Sodium: 0.2 g

Fibre: 1.2 g

Tomato Salsa √

450 g/1 lb ripe tomatoes, skinned and
    seeded
1 small onion, peeled and finely chopped
2 green chillies, seeded and diced
1 tbsp wine vinegar
freshly ground black pepper
pinch sugar
2 tbsp chopped fresh coriander or parsley

1. Finely chop the tomatoes and mix with the
   remaining ingredients. This salsa will keep
   for 4 days in the refrigerator.

Variation: During the winter, canned chopped
tomatoes can be used instead of fresh ones.

Per recipe

Calories: 182

Protein: 5.7 g

Carbohydrates: 18.5 g, of which sugars = 17.7 g

Fat: 10.0 g, of which saturates = 1.4 g

Sodium: 0.1 g

Fibre: 5.2 g

Mango and Tomato Salsa √

1 medium mango
225 g/8 oz ripe tomatoes, skinned and
    seeded
1 green chilli, seeded and diced
1 tbsp chopped fresh mint
1 tbsp chopped fresh coriander
juice of 1 lime
1 tbsp olive oil
pinch sugar
freshly ground black pepper

1. Halve the mango and remove the skin and
   stone.

2. Finely chop the mango flesh and the
   tomatoes, and mix with the remaining
   ingredients. This salsa will keep for
   1–2 days in the refrigerator.

Per recipe
Calories: 266
Protein: 3.2 g
Carbohydrates: 35.2 g, of which sugars = 34.0 g
Fat: 13.4 g, of which saturates = 1.8 g
Sodium: trace
Fibre: 5.8 g

PUDDINGS

Fruit Brûlée √
Serves 2

225 g/8 oz unsweetened cooked fruit, e.g.
    apple, blackcurrants, pears, gooseberries
    and elderflowers, or rhubarb and
    cinnamon
175 g/6 oz Greek-style natural yoghurt
2 tbsp demerara sugar

1. Preheat the grill until very hot.

2. Place the fruit in ramekins, top with the
   yoghurt and sprinkle with the sugar.

3. Place the ramekins under the hot grill until
   the sugar is bubbling.

Per serving
Calories: 374
Protein: 10.6 g
Carbohydrates: 54.6 g, of which sugars = 54.6 g
Fat: 14 g, of which saturates = 8.6 g
Sodium: 0.12 g
Fibre: 3.8 g

Grilled Peaches √
Serves 2

juice and zest of 1 orange
1 star anise
small piece cinnamon stick
2 tsp demerara sugar
2 peaches, halved and stoned
120 ml/4 fl oz low-fat vanilla yoghurt, to serve

1. Put the orange juice and zest, the spices and sugar in a pan or jug suitable for microwaving, and heat until the sugar dissolves.

2. Preheat the grill to a moderate heat.

3. Place the peaches, cut-side up, on the grill rack and spoon over a little of the juice mixture. Grill for 10 minutes, basting frequently with more juice.

4. Serve warm with the cold yoghurt.

Per serving
Calories: 126
Protein: 4.5 g
Carbohydrates: 26.9 g, of which sugars = 26.5 g
Fat: 0.9 g, of which saturates = 0.4 g
Sodium: 0.06 g
Fibre: 1.7 g

Pears in Red Wine √
Serves 2

2 firm pears, halved and cored
150 ml/5 fl oz red grape juice
2 cloves
120 ml/4 fl oz low-fat natural yoghurt
ground cinnamon
4 Biscotti (see page 150), to serve

1. Put the pears in a small saucepan and pour over the juice and cloves.

2. Heat gently for about 15 minutes, turning the pears halfway through cooking. When ready, the fruit should be tender.

3. Transfer the pears to 2 serving dishes and top with the yoghurt dusted with a little cinnamon. Serve with 2 biscotti per person.

Per serving
Calories: 192 (including 2 biscotti)
Protein: 5.8 g
Carbohydrates: 37 g, of which sugars = 30.9 g
Fat: 3.4 g, of which saturates = 0.7 g
Sodium: 0.09 g
Fibre: 3.7 g

Vanilla Yoghurt Sundae √
Serves 2

6 tbsp ready-made fruit compote
200 ml/7 fl oz low-fat vanilla yoghurt
4 tbsp granola cereal, e.g. Jordans Crunchy or Waitrose Cinnamon Crunch

1. Divide the compote between 2 serving glasses or ramekins.

2. Pour over the yoghurt and top with the cereal.

Per serving
Calories: 197
Protein: 7.4 g
Carbohydrates: 33.5 g, of which sugars = 24.1 g
Fat: 4.6 g, of which saturates = 1 g
Sodium: 0.11 g
Fibre: 3.6 g

Fruit Kebabs √

Serves 2

1 medium banana
1 clementine or satsuma
1 pear
2 Biscotti (see page 150), to serve

Make these kebabs immediately before serving so that the fruit does not have time to discolour.

1. Cut the banana into bite-size pieces.

2. Segment the clementine.

3. Halve the pear, remove the core, then cut into bite-size pieces.

4. Thread the fruits alternately on to 2 skewers.

5. Serve each skewer with a biscotti.

Per serving
Calories: 89 (129 including 1 biscotti)
Protein: 1.1 g
Carbohydrates: 21.7 g, of which sugars = 20.6 g
Fat: 0.3 g, of which saturates = 0.1 g
Sodium: none
Fibre: 2.6 g

Brioche and Red Berries √
Serves 2

50 g/2 oz raspberries
50 g/2 oz strawberries
50 g/2 oz blueberries
100 ml/3½ fl oz red fruit juice, e.g. grape, blackcurrant or cranberry

2 thick slices of brioche or 1 individual brioche cut into 4 slices
2 tsp clear honey

1. Put the berries in a saucepan with the juice and cook for 10 minutes over a moderate heat. The berries should break down a little and soften.

2. Toast the brioche slices on both sides, then spread with honey and place on a serving dish.

3. Top with the berries and serve at once.

Per serving
Calories: 138
Protein: 2.8 g
Carbohydrates: 23.9 g, of which sugars = 15.4 g
Fat: 4.2 g, of which saturates = 1.7 g
Sodium: 0.08 g
Fibre: 1.7 g

Strawberry Coeur à la Crème √
Serves 2

100 g/4 oz low-fat soft white cheese
100 g/4 oz Greek-style natural yoghurt
½ tsp vanilla essence
6 ripe strawberries, diced
1 egg white
25 g/1 oz caster sugar or sieved icing sugar

You will need special heart-shaped moulds with a perforated base for this recipe, which is best made a couple of hours before serving. Strictly speaking, the moulds should be lined with muslin as this helps the desserts to keep their shape when unmoulded, but it's up to you whether you bother with this detail.

1. Beat together the cheese, yoghurt and vanilla essence, or whizz in a blender.

2. Transfer to a mixing bowl and fold in the strawberries.

3. Whisk the egg white until it forms a light foam, then whisk in the sugar until it becomes a stiff foam.

4. Using a metal spoon, fold the foam into the strawberry mixture.

5. Divide the mixture between the moulds, sit them on saucers (because some juice will seep through the perforations), and refrigerate for up to 2 hours before serving.

Per serving
Calories: 162
Protein: 12.2 g
Carbohydrates: 19 g, of which sugars = 19 g
Fat: 4.6 g, of which saturates = 2.9 g
Sodium: 0.09 g
Fibre: 0.4 g

Mango Sorbet √
Makes 8 scoops

2 ripe mangoes, weighing a total of 600 g/
   1 lb 5 oz
juice of 1 orange
2 tbsp caster sugar
150 ml/5 fl oz hot water
2 egg whites

1. Peel the mangoes, slice the flesh from the stone and place in a liquidiser or food processor with the orange juice. Blend to a purée.

2. Dissolve the sugar in the water and pour on to the purée.

3. If you have a sorbetière or ice-cream machine, whisk the egg whites at this point until they form stiff peaks, then fold them into the purée. Transfer to the sorbetière to freeze. When frozen, spoon into a lidded container and store in the freezer.

4. If you do not have a sorbetière, pour the fruit purée into a shallow container and place in the freezer until almost frozen.

5. Whisk the egg whites until they form stiff peaks.

6. Remove the purée from the freezer and mash with a fork.

7. Fold in the whisked egg white, then return to the container and freeze for a couple of hours before serving (2 scoops per person).

Per serving (2 scoops)
Calories: 125
Protein: 2.5 g
Carbohydrates: 30.2 g, of which sugars = 29.8 g
Fat: 0.3 g, of which saturates = 0.0 g
Sodium: 0.03 g
Fibre: 3.9 g

Fresh Figs with Raspberry Coulis √

Serves 2

175 g/6 oz raspberries
1 tbsp grenadine or cranberry juice
6 fresh figs
6 tsp low-fat crème fraîche
4 Biscotti (see page 150), to serve

1. Put the raspberries and grenadine in a liquidiser and blend to a purée.

2. Slice a cross in the top of each fig, cutting almost down to the base, and insert 1 teaspoon of crème fraîche into each fruit.

3. Place three figs on each serving plate and pour the coulis around them. Serve with the biscotti.

Per serving (including 2 biscotti)
Calories: 157
Protein: 4.7 g
Carbohydrates: 27 g, of which sugars = 21 g
Fat: 4.2 g, of which saturates = 1 g
Sodium: 0.05 g
Fibre: 4.2 g

Hot Fruit Salad √

Serves 2

50 g/2 oz dried pears
50 g/2 oz dried peaches
50 g/2 oz dried apricots
50 g/2 oz prunes
50 g/2 oz raisins
1 cinnamon stick
2 cloves

2 whole green cardamoms
juice of 1 lemon
water, to cover

1. Put all the ingredients in a saucepan and slowly bring to simmering point.

2. Cook until the fruit is plump and softened – about 15 minutes.

Per serving
Calories: 277
Protein: 3.8 g
Carbohydrates: 68 g, of which sugars = 68 g
Fat: 0.8 g, of which saturates = 0.2 g
Sodium: 0.03 g
Fibre: 8.2 g

Strawberry and Amaretti Crunch √

Serves 2

6 amaretti biscuits
12 ripe strawberries, chopped
120 g/4½ oz Greek-style yoghurt

1. Roughly crush the amaretti. Set aside a few bits for garnish, but mix the rest with the fruit and yoghurt.

2. Divide the mixture between 2 serving dishes.

3. Sprinkle the reserved crumbs on top and eat immediately before the biscuits become soggy.

Per serving
Calories: 175
Protein: 5.7 g

Carbohydrates: 23.3 g, of which sugars = 12.3 g

Fat: 7.2 g, of which saturates = 4.1 g

Sodium: 0.13 g

Fibre: 1.1 g

Grilled or Barbecued Fruits √
Serves 4

1 medium pineapple

3 large pears, quartered and cored

3 large bananas, halved horizontally, then
   lengthways

2 tbsp orange juice

1 tbsp clear honey

1. Preheat the grill or barbecue to a moderate
heat.

2. Prepare the fruit and place on the grill rack.
(Sit them on a sheet of aluminium foil if using
a barbecue.)

3. Combine the orange juice with the honey.

4. If grilling the fruit, pour half the juice over
them and grill for 5 minutes. Turn the fruit,
add the remaining juice and grill for another 5
minutes.

5. If barbecuing the fruit, pour all the juice over
them and cook for about 10 minutes, turning
frequently.

Per serving

Calories: 221

Protein: 2.2 g

Carbohydrates: 54.5 g, of which sugars = 52.4 g

Fat: 0.8 g, of which saturates = 0.1 g

Sodium: 0.01 g

Fibre: 6.4 g

CAKES AND BISCUITS

Rock Cakes √
Makes about 10

225 g/8 oz wholemeal flour

1 tsp mixed spice

1 tsp baking powder

75 g/3 oz soft vegetable margarine

75 g/3 oz demerara sugar

150 g/5 oz raisins

grated rind of ½ lemon

1 egg

2 tbsp skimmed milk

1. Preheat the oven to 220°F/425°C/Gas
mark 7 and lightly oil a baking sheet.

2. Sift the flour, spice and baking powder into a
mixing bowl, returning the bran from the sieve.

3. Rub in the margarine.

4. Stir in the sugar, fruit and lemon rind.

5. Beat the egg and milk together and work into
the dry ingredients to make a light, soft dough.

6. Place forkfuls of dough on the baking sheet
and roughen the surface slightly. Bake for
15–18 minutes. (When cooled, these cakes
freeze well.)

Per cake

Calories: 200

Protein: 4 g

Carbohydrates: 33.2 g, of which sugars = 18.9 g

Fat: 7.3 g, of which saturates = 1.6 g

Sodium: 0.14 g

Fibre: 2.3 g

Almond and Pistachio Biscotti √

Makes about 40

150 g/5 oz plain white flour
100 g/4 oz golden caster sugar
1 tsp baking powder
50 g/2 oz whole almonds, roasted and
　　roughly chopped
25 g/1 oz pistachios, roughly chopped
grated rind and juice of ½ orange
grated rind of 1 lemon
1 large egg
¼ tsp vanilla essence

1. Preheat the oven to 190ºC/375ºF/Gas mark
   5 and grease a baking sheet.

2. Mix the flour, sugar and baking powder in a
   bowl.

3. Stir in the nuts and the grated orange and
   lemon rind.

4. Lightly beat in the egg and add the vanilla
   essence.

5. Drop spoonfuls of the mixture in two rows
   on the greased baking tray and shape into
   fingers 3 cm/1¼ in wide.

6. Bake for 15 minutes until golden.

7. Remove from the oven and slice each finger
   diagonally into pieces 1 cm/½ in wide.

8. Reduce the oven temperature to
   150ºC/300ºF/Gas mark 2 and return the
   biscuits to the oven for a further 10
   minutes.

9. Remove, allow to cool and store in an
   airtight tin.

Per biscotti

Calories: 37
Protein: 0.9 g
Carbohydrates: 5.8 g, of which sugars = 2.9 g
Fat: 1.2 g, of which saturates = 0.1 g
Sodium: 0.02 g
Fibre: 0.2 g

Chapter 7
Keeping weight off

This final chapter presents a selection of tried and tested ways to regulate your weight. Pick and choose to find the strategies that suit your lifestyle and circumstances.

Once you have lost weight, your body needs fewer calories than it did when you were carrying around your extra bulk. In terms of calories, you need to eat 150 less per day for every 6.5 kg/1 stone you lost.

This amounts to one less per day of any of the following:
- 1 packet of crisps (30 g/1¼ oz)
- 1 small bar of chocolate (28 g/1 oz)
- 1 lager (600 ml/1 pint)
- 1 large glass of wine (175 ml/6 fl oz)
- 1 tall full-fat milk latte or cappuccino (350 ml/12 fl oz)
- 25 g/1 oz peanut butter
- 25 g/5 tsp sugar
- 35 g/1¼ oz toffees
- 2 large biscuits

That's manageable, isn't it?

As your metabolic rate adjusts and you gradually become more active, you will not need to count calories. Your lifestyle and healthy eating habits will look after your weight. When you have finished your diet, there is no need to weigh yourself more than once a week; eventually, you can weigh yourself just once every other month. Between times the tightness of your clothes will make you aware of any extra pounds and you will adjust your eating and exercise accordingly.

SNACKING

One person's snack is another person's main meal, so it's difficult to define what constitutes a snack. In general it applies to any food eaten between meals.

Snacks account for about one quarter of our total calorie intake, so they can have a huge influence on weight. If the snacks are high in calories and no adjustment is made to food and drink intake at other times of the day, there will inevitably be some weight gain. If less is eaten at main meals to compensate, the snacks need not cause weight problems. In fact, studies have shown that lean people tend to be frequent snackers.

GRAZING

Like snacking, grazing can help regulate weight, if you do it properly. The secret is to eat little and often so that your metabolic rate (see page 97) rises and burns up food intake more efficiently. Eating four to six small meals a day rather than two or three big ones keeps your metabolism running steadily at a higher rate and prevents the peaks and troughs associated with long gaps between meals.

While grazing allows you to burn more calories, you need to be aware that you might eat more calories than you need if you are eating more frequently. At the end of the day, losing weight comes down to watching your total calorie intake – and stepping up that physical activity.

HOLDING BACK AND LETTING GO

In a world of plenty it takes a degree of restraint to prevent weight problems and obesity. Unless you are totally uninterested in food, you will spend more time telling yourself 'No' than 'Yes' when confronted with food just about everywhere you go.

Experts are still learning about how non-overweight individuals cope with food choices.

So far it seems that those who are best at controlling their weight practise a kind of 'flexible restraint', giving in to temptation now and again so that they don't feel permanently deprived.

People who have weight problems, or who regularly 'diet', have a more rigid approach to food, either saying 'No' constantly, or having episodes of bingeing. This latter habit is far more likely to lead to weight gain. Indeed, binge eating tends to be more common among obese people.

The best strategy is to stay relaxed around food: enjoy it without denying yourself, set realistic weight loss goals and exercise just enough restraint to keep things in balance.

READY-MADE MEALS

Sixty per cent of the food we eat in the UK is prepared outside the home; this figure includes convenience foods and ready-made meals.

Since healthy eating targets were set in the early 1990s, the amount of fat eaten in the average UK diet has hardly fallen at all. It currently stands at 37 per cent, so if, like most people, you are sedentary, you are eating 12 per cent more than you need. However, if you are very active, you could eat 35 per cent of your calories as fat, in which case you need to cut down by only 2 per cent. The latest figures suggest we are getting 15 per cent of our energy from saturated fat (the ideal is 10 per cent or less). As ready-made or convenience meals comprise more than half our food, it is clear that they are contributing to the weight and health problems of the nation.

If your lifestyle is such that you have to eat ready-made foods, choose those that contain no more than 5 per cent fat (read the nutrition information on the packaging); this percentage is equivalent to approximately 14 g of fat in a main meal. Choose from the 'healthy options' devised by many of the retailers and check the number of calories per serving in the product – the lower the better.

Finally, tell manufacturers, retailers and your MP that you want all food to be labelled, including items sold loose and food sold in restaurants and pubs. You especially want to see fat and calorie content, and you want food to be less calorie-dense.

EATING OUT

About 25 per cent of food is eaten outside the home, and that's a conservative estimate. However much you eat away from home now, it's likely you will do so even more in future because that is the trend. This is not in itself a bad thing: the problem with eating out is that we are not choosing healthy, low-fat foods, despite making greater efforts to do so at home. Or maybe there are not enough lower-fat, healthier options to choose from?

Most of the research on this subject has been conducted in the USA, where it has been shown that people who eat out most often tend to have a higher BMI than those who eat more frequently at home. That's because the food on sale outside the home, whether fast food or haute cuisine, is mainly high in fat. It doesn't have to be like that. In Asian countries, where eating outside the home, particularly from street vendors, is a long-standing tradition, there is no association between weight gain and eating out. That's because their fast food is stir-fried vegetables, noodles in broth or simple rice dishes, while ours is more likely to be burgers, chips and even deep-fried Mars bars!

The choice you must make comes down to fresh and healthy versus fatty and lethal. It's no contest really, is it? So ignore the marketing ploys of 'Buy one get one free', 'Eat as much as you like for next to nothing' and other such devices to deposit a load of lard into your arteries. The cost is always greater than advertised.

O-DEAR, O-BESITY
The increase in portion sizes both inside and outside the home must be one of the biggest causes of weight gain in the developed world. Of course, fast-food outlets take pride in their monster servings, and it's hard to resist offers of double helpings for just a few pence more.

Larger portion sizes have contributed to the explosion of obesity in the USA, a problem that is now manifesting itself in the UK. Go to a burger bar and you are offered 'supersized' servings, while pizza outlets encourage you to buy a large one and get a second one 'free'. Similarly, many supermarkets have increased the size of their ready-made meals to appeal to their customers' sense of value for money, and so-called 'meal deals' encourage you to buy two or three items (usually high in fat and sugar), such as a sausage roll plus crisps and chocolate, and you get a 'free' fizzy drink.

Confectionery bars are also going 'king size',

or being replaced by a large tub of mini bars, and who can eat only one? They might look small and insignificant, but before you know it, you have eaten more fat, sugar and calories than you would have done with the original size bar.

The net effect of all these selling strategies is that you eat more than you want or need, and that leads to...

UNWITTING WEIGHT GAIN
While appearing to be your friends, food manufacturers and retailers are not doing you any favours with their special offers. Larger portions are created with cheap fillers, such as

FAST AND FATTENING

Snack	Size	Grams	Cals
Burger King	Single burger		290
	XL Double whopper		873
	Small fries		250
	Large fries		490
Crisps	Standard	25	131
	Big Eat	55	289
KitKat	4 fingers	58	287
	Chunky	77	403
Maltesers	Standard	37	179
	King size	58.5	283
Mars bar	Standard	62.5	281
	Big One	85	382
Snickers	Standard	64.5	323
	Big one	100	500
Twix	Standard	58	287
	King size	85	421
Yorkie	Original	70	370
	King size	85	449

Source: British Dietitic Association (2002)

sugar and lard, so they are just fuelling you on your way to a weight problem or a heart attack. And the extra salt in that larger portion makes you want a fizzy drink, which brings more weight gain and the additional problem of dental caries. There's only one winner in this vicious cycle, and it isn't you.

NO SUCH THING AS A FREE MEAL

'Free meal' experiments done by nutritional scientists famously show that most people are 'plate cleaners' whether they are presented with a substantial 500 g/18 oz portion or a giant 1000 g/36 oz portion. It's not that they need the larger portion, because when asked to evaluate how hungry they feel after the meal, the smaller size does not leave them hungry.

Interestingly, even flexible eaters, who practise restraint much of the time and let go only occasionally, eat more when given the larger portion. However, they often leave some on the side of the plate, or adjust their next meal to compensate for over-indulging earlier. But many people do not exercise this sort of balance in their eating habits.

THE LOWDOWN ON LOW-FAT FOODS

Low-fat foods and lower-fat alternatives have been available for years, and they fund a highly profitable sector of the food industry. Nonetheless, people continue to get fatter, so it's tempting to draw the conclusion that low-fat food doesn't work.

But that is not the case. It has been proved that a reduced-fat diet results in reduced

POLLUTING EFFECT OF FOOD

If you are used to thinking of environmental pollution in terms of exhaust fumes, litter, waste incineration, cigarette smoke or industrial effluent, think again. According to sociologists, food can be a pollutant too. Obesity and weight problems are being driven by obesogenicity – namely, too much of the wrong sort of food in environments that discourage physical activity. This applies to schools, homes, workplaces and restaurants, and is compounded by over-reliance on cars, labour-saving machinery and passive recreation. Welcome to the lazy and overfed population of the obesogenic 21st century.

weight. However, the fact remains that in some countries, such as the UK and the USA, the percentage of fat in the diet has decreased at the same time as obesity has increased. Some observers have dubbed this the 'American paradox', but it affects countries around the world. Often these people are critics of lower-fat diets.

One explanation for the (putative) paradox is that people participating in dietary surveys under-report the amount of fat they eat. Another explanation could be that people eat less fat, but compensate for the reduction in calories by eating more carbohydrates. Overloading with calories from any source produces the same result: excess body fat.

The American paradox is probably also fuelled by the fact that advertisements for 'low-fat' foods give the impression that they are helpful in achieving weight loss. In truth, the opposite can be the case: what they cut down in fat, they make up in other ways. Cereal bars and breakfast cereals, for example, may contain less fat than their full-fat counterparts, but both often have large amounts of added sugar, so they ultimately contain the same number of calories. You can of course enjoy these foods if the overall balance of your diet is good; just don't be fooled into thinking that low-fat food is the same thing as low-calorie food.

When you are out shopping and want to make healthier choices, look for the following in food products:

Low total fat: 1.5–3g (or less) per 200 g of the product

Low saturated fat: less than 1.5 g per 100 g

Low sugar: less than 5 g per 100 g

Low salt: 0.12 g of sodium per 100 g

High fibre: more than 3 g of fibre per 100 g

CALORIE-LADEN COFFEE

Starbucks, Café Nero, Prêt à Manger, Café Costa – walk down any city street and you are never more than a few steps away from a coffee shop. So are they making a big, frothy, chocolate-dusted contribution to weight gain and undermining weight maintenance? Look what happens when you have regular milky coffees in addition to your daily calorie needs.

- You could put on 450 g/1 lb of fat in seven days if you drink just one full-fat large latte a day for seven days.
- You could gain 450 g/1 lb of body fat in nine

STARBUCKS CAPPUCCINO

Calories	Short	Tall	Grande	Venti
Non-fat milk	55	83	110	138
Soya milk	50	75	100	125
Full-fat milk	90	135	180	225
Fat (g)				
Non-fat milk	0	0	0	0
Soya milk	2.5	3.8	5.0	6.3
Full-fat milk	4.5	6.8	9.0	11.3

STARBUCKS LATTE

Calories	Short	Tall	Grande	Venti
Non-fat milk	80	120	160	200
Soya milk	75	113	270	188
Full-fat milk	135	208	270	338
Fat (g)				
Non-fat milk	0.5	0.8	1.0	1.3
Soya milk	4.0	6.0	8.0	10.0
Full-fat milk	7.0	10.5	14	17.5

Extras
- Whipped cream topping: 28 calories + 8.8 g fat
- 1 tsp sugar adds 20–30 calories, depending whether it's scant or heaped.
- Chocolate dust: stop right now – worrying about this is plain paranoid.

days if you drink two semi-skimmed grande cappuccinos every day.

One large, full-fat milk cappuccino contains the same calories as three fingers of KitKat, three small chocolate chip cookies or custard creams, or one 40 g packet of crisps. Then there's the fat… Two semi-skimmed big cappuccinos every day for nine days provide 86 g/3¼ oz of fat. To put that in context, women should eat no more than 70 g/2¾ oz of fat a day, and men no more than 90 g/3½ oz.

'Wait!' I hear you cry. 'I don't want to give up my coffee.' You don't have to. Coffee is not being singled out here as a 'fattening' food or drink. The point is that habitual consumption of extras – coffee, muffins, second helpings or whatever – can add up to weight gain.

One solution is to swap full-fat cappuccino and lattes for 'skinny' ones made with skimmed milk. Alternatively, if you don't need the milk for its calcium content, drink espresso or Americano because there are no calories in black coffee.

You could drink a tall cappuccino or a short latte made from skimmed milk every day for a month before you put on 450 g/1 lb of fat, and if you adjusted your food intake throughout the day to take account of the fat and calories in your daily coffee, you need never put on an ounce.

CAN ALCOHOL MAKE YOU FAT?

In theory, yes. Calories from alcohol are burned off before any other calories, so alcohol 'spares' fat from being used up. As the body prefers to store fat than other foods, such as carbohydrates and protein, alcohol has the potential to promote fat deposits and therefore weight gain.

In practice, it's unclear whether drinking alcohol is more likely to result in obesity, but it is linked to weight gain in men (think beer bellies, although I understand if you would rather not), but not among women. However, there is an argument that weight gain is due not to the alcohol itself but to the crisps, pork scratchings and peanuts that accompany it,

CALORIES IN ALCOHOL

Drink	Calories
White wine, 8.5% (125 ml/4 fl oz)	80
White or red wine, 11–13% (125 ml/4 fl oz)	104–122
Red wine, 15% (125 ml)	136
Dry cider (600 ml/1 pint)	202
Vintage cider, 10.5% (600 ml/1 pint)	566
Draught lager (600 ml/1 pint)	160–240
Draught beer (600 ml/1 pint)	180–360
Shandy (600 ml/1 pint)	150
Guinness (600 ml/1 pint)	200
Gin, vodka, whisky or other spirit, 40% (25 ml/1 fl oz)	55

and the curry, chips, kebabs or burgers that often follow a night at the pub. You get around 250 calories from a large packet of fancy crisps or 50 g/2 oz of peanuts, compared with around 160 calories from a pint of beer. A beer belly is therefore more to do with lifestyle than beer.

On a more positive note, beer does contain some useful nutrients. In fact, 1.2 litres/2 pints of beer can contain 300 mg of folate, the equivalent amount being found in a small serving of broccoli, 1.2 litres/2 pints of milk or 300 g/11 oz of fresh tomatoes. Beer also contains vitamin B_6, which works with folates to help prevent heart disease. But of course the vegetable sources of these nutrients are the better for you (sorry!).

Alcohol has another potential way of making you put on weight. The aperitifs that precede a meal stimulate the appetite and 'disinhibit' normal appetite restraints. In other words, alcohol relaxes us and makes us forget to regulate our eating. Studies show that more calories are eaten when alcohol is taken before and during a meal.

Now that the Weight Watchers organisation has put its name to a Riesling wine, the idea that alcohol converts into calories might take a firmer root in the consciousness. Riesling is a light white wine, lower in calories than many others because it contains less alcohol. Typically, table wine contains 11.5–13.5%, but the Riesling chosen by Weight Watchers contains only 8.5%.

THINK YOURSELF THIN

Sports psychologists use visualisation techniques to help teams and individuals win. They have a vision of how they are going to play, they see themselves playing winning shots, being full of energy, going the distance, crossing the line first. Of course, they train and do all the technical stuff needed for their sport, but often it is the self-belief, confidence and attitude that makes them winners.

The same principle can be applied to losing weight. You visualise yourself at the weight you want to be, you believe in your ability to achieve that and you become that person. You want to be slimmer, fitter and healthier, so you make choices about what you eat and how active you are to achieve your goal. This also applies to keeping off any weight that has been lost.

Effective visualisers think twice about whether they are really hungry before they eat. They don't automatically have a pudding when they eat out, and never order one before they have eaten the main course. They make sure water is their first choice of drink at home and at work, and don't overdo the alcohol. They don't go shopping for food when they are hungry; they plan ahead and use a shopping list. They deal with stress by relaxing through physical activity, spending time outdoors or meditating rather than relying on comfort food, alcohol or smoking. They don't weigh themselves every day or week – they go by how they feel and look in their clothes. They look forward to exercise because they choose physical activities they enjoy. They choose the stairs in the department store rather than the lift or escalator. They look for social activities and events that include physical activity.

In other words, good visualisers are active and proactive in every aspect of their lifestyle and attitude. They choose healthier options because they want the best for themselves and they deserve it.

SO WHERE DO YOU GO FROM HERE?

Since you are not able to leave Earth and go on an intergalactic search for a planet with a collective consciousness that has evolved beyond obesogenicity, your next best defence is to prevent yourself disappearing up your own vortex of spiralling weight gain.

As you know by now, to lose weight and avoid gaining weight your calories in have to equal calories out. Any excess end up as body fat. If you eat the right number of portions per day (see opposite), you can avoid the traps. Continue with your low-fat pattern of eating and make the healthy eating pyramid (see page 43) the basis of your long-term eating habits.

LOSE WEIGHT AND KEEP IT OFF

The following guidelines will help you to lose weight and not regain it. For portion sizes, see page 120.

WOMEN – TO LOSE WEIGHT

Eat around 1200 calories a day made up of the following:

- at least 5 portions of fruit and vegetables
- 6 portions of starchy carbohydrates (potatoes, pasta, rice or other grains)
- 2 portions of low-fat dairy products
- 1½ portions low-fat meat, fish or vegetarian protein
- 1–2 portions of fats
- 1 small fatty/sugary treat

WOMEN – TO MAINTAIN WEIGHT

Eat around 1700 calories a day made up of the following:

- 6–7 portions of fruit and vegetables
- 8–9 portions of starchy carbohydrates (potatoes, pasta, rice or other grains)
- 2–3 portions of low-fat dairy products
- 2 portions low-fat meat, fish or vegetarian protein
- 2 portions of fats
- 1 small fatty/sugary treat

MEN – TO LOSE WEIGHT

Eat around 1700 calories a day, as outlined in the 1700-calorie diet on page 112.

MEN – TO MAINTAIN WEIGHT

Eat around 2000 calories a day made up of the following:

- 7 portions of fruit and vegetables
- 10–11 portions of starchy carbohydrates (potatoes, pasta, rice or other grains)
- 3 portions of low-fat dairy products
- 2–3 portions of low-fat meat, fish or vegetarian protein
- 2–3 portions of fats
- 2 fatty/sugary treats

Appendix 1

Your Goal for Perfect Nutritional Health

Nutrients and other factors, such as NSPs or fibre, can be expressed as a percentage of our daily food (energy/calorie) intake. According to the World Health Organisation, countries that eat a typical Western diet could do better in a lot of areas, and the information that follows shows the percentage (in **bold**) we should be aiming for.

NUTRIENT	CALORIE GOAL	
	lower limit	upper limit
Total fat	15%	**30%**
Saturated fats	0%	**10%**
Trans fats	0%	**1%**
Polyunsaturated fats	6%	10%
Of which, omega-6 fatty acids	5%	8 %
omega-3 fatty acids	1%	2%
Monounsaturated fats	by difference*	
Total carbohydrate	**55%**	75%
Free sugars	0%	**10%**
Total fibre	not less than 25 g/1 oz a day from food	
NSPs not less than 20g/ ¾ oz a day from food		
Protein	10%	15%
Cholesterol	not more than 300 mg a day	
Salt	0 g	5 g
	(equivalent to 2 g of sodium)	
Fruits and vegetables	at least 400 g/14 oz a day	

* See Monounsaturated fats (opposite page)

Source: *Diet, Nutrition and the Prevention of Chronic Disease*, WHO (2003)

FAT

Most of the fat we eat is hidden in processed foods, meat and dairy products, pastries, snack foods and so on. While we have cut down on visible fats in spreads, and reduced fat in the foods we consume at home by swapping to skimmed milk and cutting fat off meat, we have not yet reduced fat in other ways (in main meals, biscuits, cakes and snacks), so we still get around 37 per cent of our calories from fat.

Saturated fats

Most of the saturated fat we eat comes from meat products, such as sausages, pies, burgers, ready-made meals and fried products. We also get a lot from biscuits, cakes and high-fat dairy foods, especially milk and butter. The fats used by food manufacturers to make foods often contain vegetable fats that have been fully or partially hydrogenated (hardened), which makes them high in saturated fat. Cooking fats are similarly high in saturates. Spreads generally account for a smaller part of saturated fat intake, depending on the type chosen. See also trans fats below.

Trans fats

Found in all the same foods as saturated fats,

trans fats are even worse because they raise levels of harmful cholesterol.

Polyunsaturated fats

Some vegetable oils and spreads contain both these important polyunsaturated fatty acids (PUFAs). Omega-6 is found in sunflower and soya oils, green leafy vegetables and certain nuts. Omega-3 is found in fish oils (from mackerel, herring, salmon, etc.) and plant foods, such as walnuts, rapeseed and flax oil.

Monounsaturated fats

If the 15–30 per cent of fat in your diet is not met from other fats, you can make up the difference with monounsaturates. These are found in olive oil, groundnut oil and rapeseed oil and some of their products, plus nuts and avocados.

CARBOHYDRATE

The healthier choice of foods that are predominantly carbohydrate are starches, such as rice, potatoes, pasta, bread, cassava, yam and sweet potato. If buying products made from them, choose wholegrain versions whenever possible.

Free sugars

This means the sugar added to foods by manufacturers, cooks or consumers, plus sugars naturally present in honey, syrups and fruit juices. In other words, it's the white or brown crystals in the sugar bowl. Since free sugars are regarded as 'empty calories' because they do not contribute any nutrients (vitamins, minerals or NSP), and they can also damage teeth, an upper limit has been put on consumption in a healthy diet.

FIBRE

An exact goal for fibre intake is not possible, says the WHO, because the best definition of fibre has not yet been established. However, following the recommended intake of whole-grain cereals and fruit and vegetables will provide daily 25 g/1 oz of total dietary fibre, and 20 g/¾ oz of non-starchy polysaccharides (NSPs). NSP is the collective name for certain types of fibre found in whole grains, pulses and some fruit and vegetables. The current dietary recommendation of NSPs per day in the UK is 18 g/½ oz. All types of fibre are found in wholegrain complex carbohydrates (starchy) foods, pulses fruit and vegetables.

PROTEIN

Fish, lean meat and vegetarian alternatives, such as tofu and Quorn.

CHOLESTEROL

Found mainly in shellfish, eggs, fatty meat and dairy foods. It is not really necessary to 'count' the cholesterol in your diet unless your doctor advises it.

SALT

Found in the salt cellar and added during cooking; also added to hams, bacon and cheese. Although levels in these foods cannot be reduced, manufacturers could reduce the salt content in all ready-prepared meals, canned vegetables, snack foods, bread, breakfast cereals, sauces and so on.

FRUITS AND VEGETABLES

This amount is equivalent to at least five portions of fruit and vegetables a day. Choose as wide a variety as possible.

Appendix 2

Dietary reference values (DRVs) for the UK

These are the amounts of vitamins and minerals that are used as a measure of whether the population's diet as a whole is adequate. They are not amounts designed for so-called 'optimum' nutrition. However, they are used by nutritionists to work out the needs of people with average, high and low requirements – that's why there are three sets of figures.

Estimated Average Requirement (EAR) – the average nutrient need of most people: some will need more and some less.

Reference Nutrient Intake (RNI) – the amount of a nutrient considered enough (it is actually more than enough) for most individuals, even those with high needs. If you are consuming the RNI of a nutrient, you are unlikely to be deficient.

Lower Reference Nutrient Intake (LRNI) – the amount of a nutrient considered enough for the small number of people with low needs. Most people who eat this amount will, over time, become deficient.

Some nutrient DRVs, such as vitamins B_1 and B_3, are worked out according to calorie intake, while others, such as vitamin B_6, are worked out according to how much protein is eaten. In these cases, average adult requirements are shown in the tables that follow.

Key
M = male; F = female
mg = milligrams; mcg = micrograms

DRV for vitamin A (or retinol equivalent)

Age	micrograms (mcg) per day		
	LRNI	EAR	RNI
0–12 months	150	250	350
1–6 years	200	300	400
7–10 years	250	350	500
11–14 years	250	400	600
15+ years (M/F)	300/250	500/400	700/600
Pregnant women	+100	+100	+100
Breastfeeding women	+350	+350	+350

Sources: 80 g/3¼ oz liver = 9200 mcg; 80 g/ 3¼ oz carrots = 1600 mcg; 80 g/3¼ oz spinach = 530 mcg; 1 slice Canteloupe melon = 295 mcg; 2 apricots = 200 mcg; 20 g/¾ oz watercress = 100 mcg; 1 tomato = 85 mcg; 150 g /5 oz mackerel =78 mcg; 1 boiled/ poached egg = 77 mcg; 1 tsp margarine or spread = 63 mcg

Other good food sources are dark green and orange vegetables (because the body converts their carotene content into vitamin A) and meat.

DRV for vitamin B₁ (thiamin)

Age	mg per 1000 calories		
	LRNI	EAR	RNI
0–12 months	0.20	0.23	0.30
from 1 year	0.23	0.30	0.40
Men 19–49 years*	0.60	0.80	1.00
Women 19–49 years*	0.40	0.60	0.80

*Examples worked out at 1940 calories for women, 2550 for men

Sources: 80 g/3¼ oz lean grilled beef = 0.6 mg; 40 g/1½oz (raw weight) red kidney beans = 0.21 mg; 1 Weetabix (and similar wholegrain cereals – check labels) = 0.2 mg; 1 corn on the cob = 0.18 mg; 40 g/1½oz walnuts = 0.12 mg; 1 medium-thick slice wholemeal bread = 0.09 mg

Other good sources of thiamin are meat, nuts, pulses and whole grains.

DRV for vitamin B₂ (riboflavin)

Age	mg per day		
	LRNI	EAR	RNI
0–12 months	0.2	0.3	0.4
1–3 years	0.3	0.5	0.6
4–6 years	0.4	0.6	0.8
7–10 years	0.5	0.8	1.0
11–14 years (M/F)	0.8/0.8	1.0/0.9	1.2/1.1
15+ years (M/F)	0.8/0.8	1.0/0.9	1.3/1.1
Pregnant women	+0.3	+0.3	+0.3
Breastfeeding women	+0.5	+0.5	+0.5

Sources: 150 g/5 oz mackerel = 0.75 mg; 300 ml/10 fl oz skimmed milk = 0.6 mg; 1 bowl wholegrain fortified cereal = 0.6 mg; 1 egg = 0.24 mg; 150 g/5 oz salmon = 0.22 mg; 25 g/1 oz almonds = 0.22 mg; 40g/1½oz Cheddar cheese = 0.2 mg; 2 slices thick-cut wholemeal bread = 0.08 mg

Other good food sources of riboflavin are offal, such as liver and ox heart, fortified breakfast cereal, fish roe and yoghurt.

DRV for B₃ (niacin)

Age	mg per 1000 calories		
	LRNI	EAR	RNI
All ages	4.4	5.5	6.6
Breastfeeding women	+2.3 mg/day		
Men 19–49 years*	11.2	14.0	16.8
Women 19–49 years*	8.5	10.7	12.8

*Examples worked out at 1940 calories for women, 2550 for men

Sources: 100 g/4 oz sardines = 8 mg; 100 g/4 oz chicken = 6 mg; 40 g/1½oz fortified breakfast cereal = 4.8 mg; 25 g/1 oz peanuts or peanut butter = 3.75 mg; 2 slices wheatgerm bread = 3 mg; 2 medium slices wholemeal toast = 2.5 mg; 1 lean rasher back bacon = 1.8 mg; 300 ml/½pint draught bitter = 1.41 mg; 200 g/7 oz baked beans = 1 mg; 25 g/1 oz sunflower seeds = 0.5 mg

Other good sources of niacin are oily fish and offal, such as liver.

DRV for vitamin B₆

Age	mcg per gram of protein		
	LRNI	EAR	RNI
0–6 months	3.5	6	8
7–9 months	6	8	10
10–12 months	8	10	13
from 1 year	11	13	15
Men 19–49 years*	1.0	1.2	1.4
Women 19–49 years*	0.8	0.9	1.2

*Examples worked out at protein intake of 14.7% of total energy intake on 1940 calories for women, 2550 for men.

Sources: 40g/1½oz fortified breakfast cereal = 1 mg; 100 g/4 oz turkey = 0.6 mg; half avocado = 0.6 mg; 100g/4 oz liver = 0.5 mg; 1 medium banana = 0.5 mg; 25 g/1 oz walnuts = 0.18 mg; 80g/3½oz sweet potato = 0.17 mg; 2 lean rashers bacon = 0.14 mg; 80g/3½oz spinach = 0.14 mg; 100 g/4 oz beans (e.g. red kidney) = 0.12 mg

Other good food sources include plantain, fish and meat.

DRV for vitamin B_{12}

Age	mcg per day		
	LRNI	EAR	RNI
0–6 months	0.10	0.25	0.30
7–12 months	0.25	0.35	0.40
1–3 years	0.30	0.40	0.50
4–6 years	0.50	0.70	0.80
7–10 years	0.60	0.80	1.00
11–14 years	0.80	1.00	1.20
15+	1.00	1.25	1.50
Breastfeeding women	+0.5	+0.5	+0.5

Sources: 100 g/4 oz herring (grilled) = 8 mcg; 150 g/5 oz cod = 3 mcg; 1 boiled egg = 0.9 mcg; 300 ml/10 fl oz skimmed milk = 0.9 mcg; 10 g/¼ oz yeast extract = 0.05 mcg

As vitamin B_{12} is found mainly in meat and other animal products, vegetarians need to take special care that they get sufficient in their diet. Vegans should take supplements.

DRV for folate

Age	mcg per day		
	LRNI	EAR	RNI
0–12 months	30	40	50
1–3 years	35	50	70
4–6 years	50	75	100
7–10 years	75	110	150
11+ years	100	150	200
Pregnant women	+200	+200	+200
Breastfeeding women	+60	+60	+60

(Women who might become pregnant are advised to take daily supplements of 400 mcg or 0.4 mg folic acid.)

Sources: 3 tbsp or 1 portion whole lentils (brown, green, continental or Puy, boiled) = 216 mcg; 3 tbsp or 1 portion split or red lentils (boiled) = 102 mcg; 40 g/1½oz fortified breakfast cereal = 100 mcg; 80 g/3¼ oz spinach = 97 mcg; 80 g/3¼ oz spring greens = 88 mcg; 1 slice honeydew melon = 50 mcg; medium slices wholemeal bread = 25 mcg

Other good food sources include baked beans, beef and yeast extracts, Brussels sprouts and other green leafy vegetables, brown rice, cauliflower, eggs, green beans, oranges, parsnips, peas, potatoes, pulses, such as black-eye beans and chickpeas, white bread, wholegrain pasta and yoghurt.

DRV for vitamin C

Age	mg per day		
	LRNI	EAR	RNI
0–12 months	6	15	25
1–10 years	8	20	30
11–14 years	9	22	35
15+ years	10	25	40
Pregnant women	+10	+10	+10
Breastfeeding women	+30	+30	+30

Sources: 80 g/3¼ oz broccoli = 88 mg; half a grapefruit = 32 mg; 1 mandarin = 30 mg; 80 g/3¼ oz cooked spring greens = 20 mg; 80 g/3¼ oz grated carrot = 5 mg; 80 g/3¼ oz cherries = 4 mg; eating apple = 3 mg

Other good food sources include all citrus fruit, and fruit and vegetables in general.

DRV for vitamin D

Age	mcg per day
	RNI
0–6 months	8.5
6–3 years	7.0
4–64 years (provided skin is exposed to sun)	0
65+ years	10.0
Pregnant and breastfeeding women	+10.0

Sources: 100 g/4 oz sardines canned in tomato sauce = 7.5 mcg; 1 boiled egg = 0.96 mcg; 10 g/¼ oz butter, spread (fortified) or margarine = 0.8 mcg

Vitamin D is made mostly by the normal exposure of skin to daylight, so for most people dietary sources are not essential. However, good food sources include oily fish and fats and spreads.

DRV for vitamin E

There is no LRNI, EAR or RNI set for vitamin E, but the DRVs contain the following example based on a typical PUFA intake of 6 per cent of total energy intake: 1940 calories for women, 2550 for men.

Age	mg per day
19-49 years (M/F)	7/5

Sources: 5 g/1 tsp sunflower oil = 7.3 mg; 5 g/1 tsp polyunsaturated spread = 6 mg; 80g/31/4oz sweet potato = 4.8 mg; 25 g/1 oz walnuts = 4.5 mg; 80 g/3¼ oz blackberries = 2.8 mg; half an avocado = 2.4 mg

Other good sources include vegetable oils, other nuts, pine kernels, potato crisps, wheatgerm and green leafy vegetables.

The amount of vitamin E you need depends on how much polyunsaturated fats (PUFAs) you eat. About 0.4 mg of vitamin E is needed for every gram of polyunsaturated fat.

DRV for calcium

Age	mg per day		
	LRNI	EAR	RNI
0–12 months	240	400	525
1–3 years	200	275	350
4–6 years	275	350	450
7–10 years	325	425	550
11–14 years (M/F)	450/480	750/624	1000/800
15–18 years (M/F)	450/480	750/624	1000/800
19+ years (M/F)	400/400	525/525	700/700
Breastfeeding women	+550	+550	+550

Sources: 80 g/3¼ oz spinach = 480 mg; 25 g/1 oz Cheddar = 400 mg; 125 ml/4 fl oz low-fat yoghurt = 225 mg; 150 ml/5 fl oz skimmed milk = 195 mg; 25 g/1 oz almonds = 62 mg; 80 g/3¼ oz cooked chickpeas = 25 mg; 1 tbsp raisins = 18 mg

Other good sources include low-fat dairy foods, fortified soya milk, seeds, dried fruit, hard water and nuts. (For more dietary suggestions, see Osteoporosis, page 37.)

DRV for iron

Age	LRNI	mg per day EAR	RNI
0–3 months	0.9	1.3	1.7
4–6 months	2.3	3.3	4.3
7–12 months	4.2	6.0	7.8
1–3 years	3.7	5.3	6.9
4–6 years	3.3	4.7	6.1
7–10 years	4.7	6.7	8.7
11–18 years (M/F)	6.1/8.0*	8.7/11.4*	11.3/14.8*
19–49 years (M/F)	4.7/8.0*	6.7/11.4*	8.7/14.8*
50+ years (M/F)	4.7/4.7	6.7/6.7	8.7/8.7

*About 10 per cent of women with high menstrual losses will need more iron than shown. Their needs are best met by taking iron supplements.

Sources: 1 bowl bran flakes = 8 mg; 300 g/11 oz chilli con carne = 6.6 mg; 2 thick-cut slices wholemeal bread = 4 mg; 1 bowl cereal with fruit (e.g. raisins) = 3.5 mg; 80 g/3¼ oz lean lamb = 1.3 mg; 80 g/3¼ oz broccoli = 1 mg; 50 g/2 oz nuts and raisins = 1 mg

Other good food sources of iron include dried fruit, fortified breakfast cereal, seeds, lean red meat, offal, eggs and green leafy vegetables.

DRV for potassium

Age	mg per day LRNI	RNI
0–3 months	400	800
4–6 months	400	850
7–9 months	400	700
10–12 months	450	700
1–3 years	450	700
4–6 years	600	1100
7–10 years	950	2000
11–14 years	1600	3100
15+ years	2000	3500

Sources: 225 g/8 oz baked potato = 1420 mg; 2 tomatoes (grilled) = 420 mg; 1 banana = 400 mg; 80g/3¼ oz lean steak (grilled) = 400 mg; 150 ml/5 fl oz orange juice = 305 mg; 25 g/1 oz mixed nuts = 200 mg; 2 slices wholemeal bread = 166 mg; 80g/3¼ oz peas = 104 mg; 1 low-fat yoghurt = 95 mg

Other good sources of potassium include vegetables, fruit, dairy produce, seeds, nuts, meat, fish, wholegrain breads and cereal.

DRV for selenium

Age	mcg per day LRNI	RNI
0–3 months	4	10
4–6 months	5	13
7–9 months	5	10
10–12 months	6	10
1–3 years	7	15
4–6 years	10	20
7–10 years	16	30
11–14 years	25	45
15–18 years (M/F)	40/40	70/60
19+ years (M/F)	40/40	75/60
Breastfeeding women	+15	+15

Sources: 2–3 Brazil nuts = 100 mcg; tuna sandwich (2 slices wholemeal bread) = 59 mcg; 50 g/2 oz (dry weight) green or brown lentils = 50 mcg; 125 g/4½oz grilled salmon = 38 mcg; 25 g/1 oz mixed nuts and raisins = 42 mcg; 75 g/3 oz lean pork = 15 mcg

Other good sources are wholemeal flour and bread, nuts (cashews, walnuts), fish (tuna, swordfish, cod, sardines), shellfish (prawns, mussels), offal (liver) and sunflower seeds.

DRV for sodium

Age	LRNI	RNI
0–3 months	140	210
4–6 months	140	280
7–12 months	200	320
10–12 months	200	350
1–3 years	200	500
4–6 years	280	700
7–10 years	350	1200
11–14 years	460	1600
15+ years	575	1600

Daily sodium needs for adults are all too easily met. For example, a Pot Noodle meal contains 1.5 g of sodium – that's nearly 4 g of salt – when we should have no more than 5 g per day in total. But it could be worse, a Big Mac and large fries supplies 2.1 g sodium, equivalent to 6.25 g salt.

A typical day provides far more than we need: 40 g/1½ oz bran cereal = 0.3 g; 1 medium-thick slice white bread = 0.2 g; 200 g/7 oz baked beans = 1.1 g; 40 g/1½oz packet of crisps = 0.2 g; 1 snack salami (peperami) = 0.5 g.

DRV for zinc

Age	LRNI	mg per day EAR	RNI
0–6 months	2.6	3.3	4.0
7–3 years	3.0	3.8	5.0
4–6 years	4.0	5.0	6.5
7–10 years	4.0	5.4	7.0
11–14 years	5.3	7.0	9.0
15+ (M/F)	5.5/4.0	7.3/5.5	9.5/7.0
Breastfeeding women			
0–4 months	+6.0	+6.0	+6.0
4+ months	+2.5	+22.5	2.5

Sources: 1 oyster = 6 mg; 100 g/4 oz lean steak (grilled) = 5.6 mg; 100 g/4 oz sardines canned in tomato sauce = 2.7 mg; egg sandwich (2 slices wholemeal bread) = 2 mg; 40 g/1½ oz Edam cheese = 1.6 mg; 25 g/1 oz pumpkin seeds = 1.6 mg; tuna sandwich (2 slices multigrain bread) = 1.5 mg; 1 bowl cereal containing raisins or other dried fruit = 1.3 mg; 1 bowl porridge made with milk = 1.3 mg; 3 tbsp sweetcorn kernels = 0.5 mg

Other good sources of zinc include seafood, meat, sardines, liver, wholegrain breads and cereals, pumpkin seeds, eggs, pulses, milk, nuts and oats.

ESTIMATED AVERAGE ENERGY REQUIREMENTS (EARS)

Age	EARs calories per day/megajoules (MJ)	
	Males	Females
0–3 months	545 (2.28)	515 (2.16)
4–6 months	690 (2.89)	645 (2.69)
7–9 months	825 (3.44)	765 (3.20)
10–12 months	826 (3.85)	865 (3.61)
1–3 years	1230 (5.15)	1165 (4.86)
4–6 years	1715 (7.16)	1545 (6.46)
7–10 years	1970 (8.24)	1740 (7.28)
11–14 years	2220 (9.27)	1845 (7.92)
15–18 years	2755 (15.15)	2110 (8.83)
19–50 years	2550 (10.60)	1940 (8.10)
51–59 years	2550 (10.60)	1900 (8.00)
60–64 years	2380 (9.93)	1900 (7.99)
65–74 years	2330 (9.71)	1900 (7.96)
75+ years	2100 (8.77)	1810 (7.61)
Pregnant women*		+200 (+0.80)*
Breastfeeding women		
1 month		+450 (+1.90)
2 months		+530 (+2.20)
3 months		+570 (+2.40)
4–6 months group 1		+480 (+2.90)
4–6 months group 2		+570 (+2.40)
6 months group 1		+240 (+1.00)
6 months group 2		+550 (+2.30)

*Last trimester only

Source: Department of Health, London (1991)

Appendix 3

Glycaemic Index

As the concept of the glycaemic index (GI) is quite complex, and because many people find it difficult to apply, it is dealt with here rather than in the main text of this book.

Among those trying to lose weight and improve their diet the most important things to concentrate on initially are calories and sorting out weight problems. Only then should you go on to the second stage, which involves dealing with GI. But if you want to know a little more, read on.

The glycaemic index is a measure of the effect foods have on blood-sugar levels. Foods that have a low GI break down slowly during digestion, releasing energy gradually into the bloodstream and resulting in a smaller rise in blood sugar and a more even supply of energy. As you might expect, this is a good thing.

- It helps control hunger, appetite and weight gain.
- It improves sensitivity to insulin and helps control diabetes.
- It can possibly help prevent type 2 diabetes.
- It appears to lower raised blood-fat levels, offering protection to the heart.

Foods have a GI ranking from 0 (good) to 100 (bad). Low GI foods score 55 or below, intermediate GI foods score 55–70 and high GI foods score more than 70. Some examples of each of these appear below.

SELECTED GI FOOD RATINGS

Low GI Foods (55 or below)		Intermediate GI Foods (56–70)		High GI Foods (above 70)	
Bread: fruit loaf	47	Bread: wholegrain rye	68	Bread: English white	70
pumpernickel	41	wholewheat	69	French baguette	95
Chocolate	49	Couscous	65	Chips	75
Fish	30	Crispbread	69	Coco pops	77
Fruit:		Croissant	67	High-energy (sports)	
apples and pears	38	Digestive biscuit	59	drinks	around 95
bananas	55	Green pea soup	66	Iced biscuits	80
dried apricots	38	Honey	58	Jelly beans	80
Pasta: white &		Macaroni cheese	64	Potato: baked	80
wholemeal	32–50	Mars bar	68	Rice: short-grain	85
Porridge	42	Muesli	56	sticky rice	87
Pulses, beans and		Muffin	60	glutinous rice	98
lentils	30-40	Taco shell	68	Rice cakes	82

The GI ranking of food has caused some confusion because there have been a few surprises. For example, some breads, potatoes and rice have high GI rankings compared with ice-cream, some confectionery and a few other sugary foods that did not produce as dramatic a rise in blood sugar as had been predicted.

The GI score of potatoes and rice varies according to type and method of cooking. Baked potatoes, for example, have a high GI of 85; hot boiled potatoes have an intermediate score of 56; and cold boiled potatoes (as in potato salad) have a low GI of 50.

Similarly, good-quality pasta has a low GI factor because the durum wheat from which it is made is very hard and resists digestive enzymes, making it slower to break down and release energy. Pasta made from softer flour or rice is digested more quickly and therefore has a higher score.

Regardless of GI score, however, pasta, potatoes, rice and other starchy foods are valuable, particularly the wholemeal and wholegrain varieties.

If you are interested in finding out more about the GI ratings of foods, consult a specialist book, such as *The Glucose Revolution: GI Plus* by Jennie Brand-Miller, Kaye Koster-Powell and Anthony Leeds (Hodder & Stoughton, 2001).

Glossary

Antioxidant – a vitamin, mineral, phyto (plant) chemical or other substance that delays or prevents oxidation.

Carotenoids – pigments ranging in colour from red to orange and yellow. They are found in plant foods and plant-eating animals that humans eat for meat. There are more than 600 carotenoids, beta-carotene being the most widely available and an active antioxidant.

Coumestrol – a type of phyto-oestrogen found mainly in beansprouts.

DNA – deoxyribonucleic acid, the genetic material found in the nucleus of every cell in the body. It consists of coiled strands of 46 chromosomes in 23 pairs. When damaged, DNA may make mistakes when replicating cells, which can lead to cancer.

DPA – docosahexaenoic acid, the most valuable form of omega-3 fatty acid.

EPA – eicosapentaenoic acid, a form of omega-3 fatty acid.

Flavonoids – the largest group of 'phenolic compounds'. They act as powerful antioxidants and are widespread in fruit, vegetables and tea. The flavonoid group has many subdivisions, including isoflavones found in soya, and lignans found in whole grains, linseed and pulses. Other types of flavonoid include anthocyanis, which give cherries and blueberries their red and blue colours, flavones in tea, and flavonols in onions, apples and other fruit and vegetables.

Free-radicals – highly reactive molecules made in the body and also found in pollutants. A free radical molecule is one electron short (electrons are usually paired), so they grab an electron from another molecule, disturbing the chemical balance by making another electron a single (reactive) unit. Free radicals are produced constantly in the body and need to be 'mopped up' by antioxidants (e.g. vitamins E and C, the minerals selenium and zinc, and flavonoids) to prevent them damaging DNA (a cancer risk) or oxidising LDL cholesterol, which enables it to become plaque in the arteries.

HDL – high-density lipoprotein, a beneficial form of cholesterol.

Homocysteine – an amino acid that is a natural by-product of the breakdown of protein.

Isoflavone – see Flavonoids

LDL – low-density lipoprotein, a harmful form of cholesterol.

NSPs – non-starchy polysaccharides, the collective name for different types of fibre found in whole grains, pulses and certain fruits and vegetables, which lower cholesterol.

Oxidation – a reaction in the body between food and oxygen that produces free radicals.

Phenolic compounds – are the largest category of phyto (plant) chemicals found in fruit, vegetables, nuts and herbs, including all the flavonoids.

Phyto-oestrogens -- plant hormones found in foodstuffs such as soya, linseed and pulses. They are fermented during digestion by friendly gut bacteria to make weak forms of the female hormone oestrogen. These can also act as anti-oestrogens. By taking the place of the sex hormone oestrogen in the body, they dilute its effect, as they are very much weaker; thus they can have an anti-oestrogen effect. Both the anti-oestrogen and normal, but weaker, oestrogen effects seem to be beneficial in fighting heart disease and cancer, and probably osteoporosis.

Polysaccharides – indigestible starches (carbohydrates) in raw foods, such as potatoes and rice, which become digestible when heated or cooked with water. However, some forms of heat treatment, such as that used to make certain breakfast cereals, turn some of these starches into 'resistant starch', which is also indigestible, or less digestible, therefore acting like fibre.

VLDL – very low-density lipoprotein, a harmful form of cholesterol.

Index